ALLERGY CURES YOUR ALLERGIST NEVER MENTIONED

Sterling R. Booth, Jr.

ALLERGY CURES YOUR ALLERGIST NEVER MENTIONED

Sterling R. Booth, Jr.

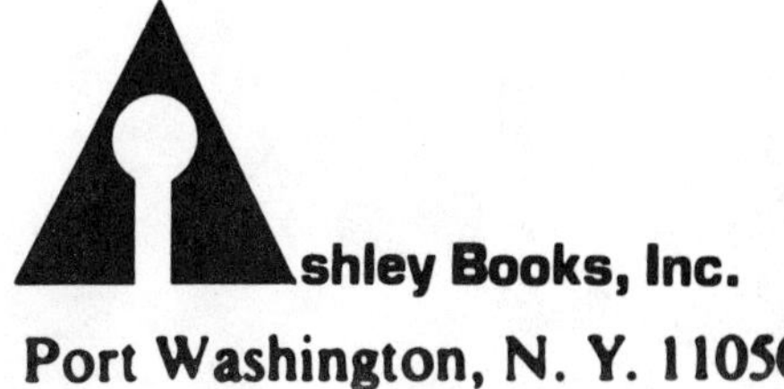

Port Washington, N. Y. 11050

This work is dedicated to my family, Mildred Louise Thomas Booth, her beloved parents Mr. and Mrs. John David Thomas, my son Sterling Rawlinson Booth III, daughters Joan Ethel Booth and Gail Elizabeth Booth Brown, son-in-law L. Edwin Brown, Jr., my guitar-picking brother Douglas Monroe Booth for his suggestions on the value of honeycomb chewing, my aunt Lois Marie Booth Ingram, my uncle Lloyd Tyler and wife Nancy McLain Tyler, as well as James H. Stephenson, M.D., whose words of encouragement and work entitled *A Doctor's Guide To Helping Yourself With Homeopathic Remedies* inspired me in no small way.

CONTENTS

FOREWORD

This interesting book of Sterling Booth's is written in the style of Mr. Jarvis of Vermont, full of pithy, practical observations drawn from the author's own experience. It is also reminiscent of Gerard and Culpepper, those empiric herbalists whose compendia were probably clutched under the arms of Mr. Booth's own ancestors when they first came to the Tidewater and Carolina area in the seventeenth and eighteenth centuries.

Thus, in the great American tradition of self-discovery and gut-knowledge, Mr. Booth carries on the work of Louis Bromfield, Bernar MacFadden, Adelle Davis, Linda Clark, Rodale father and son and, more recently, Jethro Clark. Welcome to the ranks, and may your good work continue!

James Stephenson, M.D.

Introduction

In October, 1977, the National Center for Health Statistics in Washington, D.C., reported that 567,600,000 visits were made to doctors' offices in 1975. Astonishingly, respiratory ailments accounted for 14 percent of this staggering total, or approximately 80,000,000 visits! Indeed, this single category outranked all other illnesses, including heart disease which accounted for 10 percent of the total. Almost 14,000,000 Americans are plagued annually with hay fever from pollen alone and another 6,000,000 suffer from asthma. Those classified as having bronchitis number over 6,500,000 and emphysema is becoming more common than ever before. The American Academy of Allergy estimated several years ago that about 15 percent, or in excess of 30,000,000, of the American populace can now be classified as allergy sufferers, while 47,000,000 are said by the American Lung Association to have respiratory diseases, including chronic colds.

Steady increases in various forms of industrial pollutants in the air we breathe—quite apart from the miseries wrought by pollen, dust, animal dander, mold, cigarette smoke, food or drug allergens—add to respiratory suffering on a scale never before known to mankind. Meanwhile, highly evolved medicines the human body cannot assimilate bring about side effects often worse than the original complaint. Asthmatics have been known to suffer severe seizures when given decongestants containing aspirin. The respiratory drug Isoproterenol is alleged to have killed 3,500 asthmatics in England alone. Indeed, today's so-called respiratory "wonder" drug may well become tomorrow's "blunder" drug!

I was one of those 6,000,000 Americans cursed with asthma, one of the 14,000,000 plagued by hay fever. During my years of suffering I must have tried practically all of the prescription and nonprescription drugs available. I got little if any relief. Then, through a combination of luck and persistence, I developed a program of vitamins, good nutrition, common sense, and exercise which has freed me from medication. Best of all, it has freed me from my chronic asthma, and my formerly acute hay fever is now at least 90 percent under control.

I have not taken asthma medication since February 15, 1973, or a hay fever tablet since February 28, 1973.

Once I started my program I was able to eliminate respiratory drugs in about six months without any known side effects. Although each case of asthma, hay fever, or bronchitis is different, just as each individual is different, I believe there are 'many elements of my plan that can be of benefit to all sufferers. In the chapters that follow I will describe my regimen in detail and offer suggestions which other respiratory sufferers may wish to try. In brief, my program consists of:

1. a vital food plan (including honey—the wonder food)
2. a detoxification system
3. a specially designed vitamin-mineral formula
4. what I call my "off-beat remedies"
5. the herbal approach.

It took me some time and effort to get rid of my asthma, but it was worth it. If you're fed up with expensive prescriptions, useless over-the-counter drugs, and too many visits to doctors, you may find some simple solutions in these pages.

CHAPTER I
A TIMELY DISCOVERY

In early August, 1972, I gaspingly awaited another daybreak without sleep as I lay propped on two nonallergenic pillows. During the preceding days I had received from zero to four hours of "sleep" nightly because of severe asthma. The dismal prospect of working all day amidst those nicotine-saturated, cigarette-sucking boobs at the office filled me with no small alarm. As I remained propped abed in uttermost dread of another day filled with cigarette pollution which would make my breathing difficulties worse, I suddenly recalled a conversation I had a few months earlier while visiting my cousin Daniel Matherson McLain. I scarcely thought then that a discussion on the reported marvels of Vitamin E (alpha tocopheryl type) could possibly lead to actions that would lengthen my own lifespan!

Despite my extreme breathing difficulty on that morning in early August, 1972, I did two things that helped me cure myself of asthma. I dizzily arose from bed and walked two miles to the office (with no small effort). I now realize that my afflictions in those agonizing times would have been worse had I not frequently walked to work. And later that day I purchased 100 capsules of Vitamin E (alpha tocopheryl). Each capsule contained 200 International Units and I began taking one capsule daily.

At the time of my Vitamin E purchase, I was taking a variety of drugs in various quantities. For example, I'd take a maximum of six asthma tablets on Monday to soothe my lower respiratory system. Then on Tuesday I would take a maximum of eight hay fever tablets in an effort to gain relief for my upper respiratory system. Often I felt it necessary to take some of both medicines on the same day when confronted with hay fever sneezing fits and suffocating asthma attacks within a relatively short span of one another. I also took great care to prevent overdosing.

When an asthma or hay fever sufferer tells his physician that he has become "immune" to his current dosages (great though they may be), the doctor is likely to either change chemical brands or increase the volume of the drugs already being prescribed. I recall all too well having started with low dosages and gradually increasing my ingestions as my condition worsened. It seemed like a never-ending progression—my condition continued to deteriorate, dosages were stepped up, yet I was no better off than before. By that August day when I started taking Vitamin E, I was beginning to wonder if all the medicines were harming me rather than helping me. Yet my system was so thoroughly imbued with medications that, notwithstanding the obvious value of Vitamin E, I felt unable to discontinue them at once. A tapering-off period thus followed, in which I cut down my intake about 30 percent between September and November, 1972; 20 percent in December, 1972; and the remaining 50 percent during January-February, 1973.

Approximately two weeks after commencing my program, I increased my daily intake of Vitamin E from 200 International Units to 400. A singularly unusual thing occurred after going to bed that night. Around midnight, I felt an unbelievable (by past standards) surge of air enter my lungs. Shortly thereafter, I increased my intake to 600 I.U.'s daily and then cautiously tested 800 I.U.'s. There was absolutely no toxic effect and on days when I suffered more than the usual "stresses" I quite profitably took three 400 I.U. capsules of Vitamin E.

Anyone tormented with bronchial asthma can appreciate my exhilaration over the surge of oxygen. During an asthma attack, a sufferer often experiences a terrifying feeling of suffocation as he struggles to exhale "stale" air and inhale "fresh" air. Apparently the doses of Vitamin E I had taken reduced stress, thus lessening the tightness in my chest and allowing the surge of air. As I lay in bed (though still propped on my two nonallergenic pillows), I rejoiced in my good fortune. The temptation to awaken Mildred, my long-suffering wife, was great but I reconsidered, fearing that my improvement was just a fluke. I fell asleep easily and slept through the night with unaccustomed comfort.

Until this incident, the only thing I could sense about Vitamin E's marvelous properties was that my legs were seemingly less tired than previously. But now it was apparent that I was pointed in the right direction and I was beginning to suspect that the methods being used by our medical school graduates to control respiratory conditions left something to be desired. In fact, I was on the verge of wondering (with all due respect) if the term *quack* did not more aptly describe some of our licensed allergy physicians than a number of the degreeless independent researchers who qualify only as "health nuts."

At present, Vitamin E is considered by many researchers essentially nontoxic if properly used with your *doctor's approval.* However, since large amounts may cause the blood pressure to rise in those not accustomed to it (and there are also those who may have undiagnosed high blood pressure), it would be wise to have your blood pressure checked before taking *any* Vitamin E. According to medical studies, those with high blood pressure (hypertension) would thus take only small amounts of Vitamin E initially and gradually increase the intake as the blood pressure is properly regulated. Dr. Wilfrid E. Shute (considered by many to be one of the world's foremost Vitamin E authorities) reportedly believes that this vitamin increases the volume of blood pumped by the heart and that too sudden a build up of Vitamin E in cases of very high blood pressure can be hazardous. The help, therefore, of a physician who knows how to utilize Vitamin E in correct amounts in special cases of high blood pressure (and chronic rheumatic heart disease where too much Vitamin E could be fatal) is essential. Diabetics too should be sure to consult their doctors before beginning a Vitamin E program since the efficacy of insulin may be affected by the vitamin.

I was soon to learn that in addition to being a definite aid to circulation and thus my breathing, Vitamin E was beginning to be widely used to protect the respiratory system against air pollution. Excessive amounts are reportedly excreted from the body and it is said that the effects of Vitamin E disappear in approximately three days. If this is true, it would be necessary for those heavily dependent upon Vitamin E to consume it regularly.

In addition to Vitamin E's highly publicized use in fighting heart disorders and as a "secret weapon" in the field of athletics, it has been reportedly used in the treatment of sundry allergies, anemia, arthritis, bruises, burns, carbuncles, cataracts, colitis, cystic fibrosis, cystitis, diabetes (with care being taken to properly regulate the insulin intake), emphysema, epilepsy, eyestrain, gangrene, gout, headaches, hemorrhoids, hypertension (with, as noted, certain precautions), hyperthyroidism, mental illness, multiple sclerosis, nephritis, numbness or cramps in the legs, osteomyelitis, Parkinson's disease, phlebitis, prostatitis, purpura, sterility, ulcers, varicose veins, warts and the hot flashes of menopause!

CHAPTER II

FORMULATING A VITAL FOOD PROGRAM

My slowly evolving success with Vitamin E therapy led me to suspect a food program could be devised that might eventually overcome my chronic asthma as well as control my acute year-round hay fever that dated from early childhood and had led to my increasingly severe bronchial difficulties.

After considerable reflection, it finally dawned on me that our early ancestors survived in large measure, according to season, upon raw unpolluted fruits, herbs, vegetables, roots or tubers, grain plants, nuts or seeds, seaweeds, eggs, honey and slain animals (much as several Eskimo tribes still consume raw blubber with no revulsion whatsoever). Moreover, it appeared likely that the basic diet was low in saturated fats, contained organic salts only, and was readily assimilable. Needless to say, white sugar, nonassimilable food additives, table salt, white bread, French fries, relishes, catsup, commercial candies, hot dogs, mustard, potato chips, pretzels, pickles, synthetic sweeteners, ice cream, soda pop, puffed rice balls, hamburgers, sausages, spaghetti, macaroni, breakfast cereals saturated with sugar and washed down with moon-orbiting Tang were unknown to our forest primeval forefathers. While our early ancestors may have run a rather goodly chance of being eaten alive while drinking spring water, they probably had a quite remarkable working knowledge of herbal medicine and ran a lesser risk of being systematically poisoned than now obtains at the corner drug store.

FOOD FOR THOUGHT: More often than not, allergens are protein in nature. If proteins are not properly digested, intestinal bacteria putrefy as a consequence and the amino acid histidine may then be converted into histamine. Histamine in turn causes nasal stuffiness, sneezing, coughing, itching, runny nose, etc. The pharmaceutical houses do a land office business in antihistamines as a result and one popular type, chlorpheniramine maleate by name, is found in at least sixty-five over-the-counter medications. High blood pressure, fatigue, drowsiness and blurred vision are among the more common side effects of some twenty-five basic chemical formulas and around one hundred brand name preparations on the market. Since an allergic individual may register any number of adverse reactions to even one decongestant preparation in due time, where does one run to find an allergist who can qualify as an expert on even one of the twenty-five basic formulas?

With all these things firmly in mind, I began to change my diet to incorporate more natural, healthful foods. I did it gradually, experimenting with different types and amounts of food until I found those that agreed with me and seemed most beneficial. Here, in the form of *suggestions,* are the foods that helped me cure my asthma. Remember to check with your doctor before changing your eating habits. And remember too that a wide range of foods is essential for good health. Eating a limited selection of foods for any period of time is not only boring but can be hazardous.

SUGGESTION 1: Eat at least TWO meals daily of raw, well-washed, fresh fruits or vegetables, regularly adding one's choice of a few unsalted, high-grade protein sunflower seeds, peanuts or almonds as a meat substitute (despite their being relatively high in calories).

Fruits and vegetables can be consumed (and chewed slowly) in various combinations according to taste and digestibility. Initially, a single, undersized banana gave me unmerciful indigestion but I was eventually able to regularly eat one, or several, with no ill effects whatever. Of course, common sense has to be exercised. For example, turnip or mustard greens are almost impossible to eat raw in quantity.

As for special "respiratory foods," virtually all raw fruits and vegetables are of gradual corrective value. Those having a high Vitamin A content (particularly unpeeled carrots and sweet potatoes) should be eaten very regularly. Freshly peeled citrus fruits (oranges, grapefruits, tangerines and tangelos) are valuable because of their high Vitamin C level as well as the bioflavonoids (Vitamin P) they contain. Bioflavonoids are found in the white, pulpy substance inside citrus fruits. Asthmatics should also take a teaspoon of squeezed lime or lemon juice several times daily between meals.

I realize that some people cannot suddenly "reprogram" their eating habits for one reason or another. Yet it is not difficult to introduce fresh, raw fruits and vegetables into the daily diet. Fresh fruit can replace calorie-laden, sugar-loaded desserts. Raw vegetables add new texture and taste to salads. Raw unsaturated cooking oils (corn, sunflower seed, etc.), lemon juice, or apple cider vinegar made from the pure juice only can be used to dress these salads. Or learn how to flavor them with such "respiratory herbs" as marjoram or oregano; basil; the seeds of caraway, dill, cumin, celery (very strong), anise, fennel, sesame or sunflower, as well as such miscellaneous health-laden items as wheat bran or germ, granola, raisins, nuts, or a little powdered kelp in lieu of salt. Other tossed salad ingredients—praised in bygone days as valuable in fighting respiratory ailments—are onions, garlic, and horseradish (though difficult to digest in quantity). Sprouted seeds can also be added.

Overweight respiratory sufferers should select foods having the lowest comparative calorie and carbohydrate contents. And those people with diverticulitis, piles, or ulcer conditions should beware such troublemakers as raw peanuts, seeds in vegetables such as cucumbers or tomatoes, and skins on fruits if so advised by their doctors.

I also realize that some people will find it hard to get used to eating raw vegetables. For them, steaming can ease the transition from overcooked to raw. Steamers of various types can be purchased at most stores for a reasonable price. In a steamer, the vegetables are not actually covered with water so the nutrients aren't washed away. Any water remaining (rich in vitamins and minerals) should be used as "soup" or for other cooking purposes.

SUGGESTION 2: Let only the THIRD daily meal consist of such high-protein items as:

broiled fish or chicken (no skin) or the low-salt dietary-shelf tuna IN MODERATE AMOUNTS. (Flesh foods are generally acid-forming if overeaten and can cause heartburn, nausea or other gastric distress which can compound the miseries of asthma.);

the milder low-salt cheeses such as American cheddar (or health store unsalted cheeses where obtainable) in restrained volume;

approximately one cup of buttermilk, yogurt or sweet acidophilus milk (believed to be a valuable new antihistamine culture) because of their calcium content and their reputed ability (as opposed to mucus-forming whole sweet milk) to destroy certain putrefactive intestinal bacteria that cause allergies, ulcers, and gout.

This meal could also include:

high-protein, vegetable-derived, meat-substitute items such as several religious orders eat instead of flesh foods (commonly found in health stores);

whole-grain breads without preservatives (sometimes containing honey) which should be stored in the refrigerator to prevent spoilage;

several soft-boiled eggs each week inasmuch as the egg is a complete protein source and has many vital nutrients (including Vitamin B12 so generally scarce in raw fruits or vegetables).

Doctors are still hotly debating the role or nonrole of eggs in heart disease, so I eat them in moderate amounts only. But I honestly believe that white sugar, junk foods, and refined flour (with its Vitamin E processed out) are just a few of the substances more likely to be hazardous to the human heart than the consumption of a few nutrient-packed eggs from time to time. I feel, however, that an overabundance of animal-derived protein (particularly flesh foods) places an undue burden on the organs of elimination, is quite often mucus-forming or acid-forming and must, therefore, be consumed in moderation by respiratory sufferers.

Another good source of nonanimal protein is dried legumes (peas or beans). To prepare them for cooking, boil them in water for approximately two minutes, fully submerged. Remove the pan from the heat and allow the legumes to soak for about an hour. (This method does away with the much longer tenderizing period utilized by those who customarily soak dried legumes in cold water for half a day or more.) Cooking is resumed after the short soaking period and fewer nutrients are lost this way.

SUGGESTION 3: Try drinking liquids one-half hour before meals or an hour or two afterwards because an excess of fluid apparently impairs the overall digestive processes. For example, liquids may be taken upon arising and a little while prior to breakfast, between meals, or in the middle of the evening.

Raw fruits and vegetables actually contain approximately 70 percent to 95 percent water in its purest form and one is not likely to suffer from dehydration if no liquids are taken during mealtimes. Undoubtedly, the water found in raw fruits or vegetables is of incomparably higher grade than our tap water which is derived from carbonate compounds, inorganic minerals, soap powders, undue commercial salts, and flavored with chlorine. Only God knows what culprits lurk in our water supply.

Unfortunately, most people cannot obtain good spring, mineral or natural well water with which to properly cleanse the system and the bottled distilled water sold in some quarters is overpriced for most consumers. Fortunately, valuable liquids may be had by pouring a little apple juice as a base into a blender and pureeing in it various combinations of vegetables and/or fruits. The resulting juice, if not consumed promptly, may be stored in the refrigerator, properly covered or capped after blending to prevent Vitamin C loss.

I not only use apple juice as a base in these mixtures because of its value in fighting respiratory malfunctions but because I have sorrowfully noted that several other juices on the market are liberally saturated with salt. I often flavor my less palatable juice combinations with nature's most remarkable sweetener—honey—and have even fortified them with powdered forms of brewer's yeast, bone meal (when my calcium intake was low), alfalfa, lecithin, rose hips, wheat germ or desiccated liver in tolerable amounts.

Carrot, cranberry, blackberry, fig, grape, pineapple, prune, and citrus juices are also of great benefit in cleansing the system of its poisonous mucus deposits. Also, don't overlook consuming a daily cup of honey-flavored herbal infusions made from either althaea (or marsh mallow) roots, coltsfoot leaves, horehound (whole herb), mullein leaves or flowers, plantain leaves and ginseng, all obtainable in health food stores. (Care must be exercised in the use of herbs. See chapter 7, especially for information on herbs as a weapon in fighting respiratory ills.)

SUGGESTION 4: Eliminate wherever possible all foods containing white sugar or salt (sodium chloride). Both apparently create metabolic imbalances and put additional strain upon an asthmatic's body. Unless specifically banned because of its high calorie content (or a diabetic condition) honey can be substituted for white sugar and nature supposedly put its own correct amounts of organic salts in raw fruits and vegetables.

Physicians sometimes place high blood pressure patients on low sodium diets of less than 300 milligrams daily. This is often a difficult diet to follow. Unfortunately, only one slice of commercially produced whole wheat bread contains 122 milligrams of sodium and similar amounts are found in rye. This makes it necessary (unless a health food store is convenient) for one to make his own bread if undue salt is to be avoided. Furthermore, an eight-ounce cup of unprocessed green peas contains a single milligram of natural, assimilable, organic salt, but the same cup of commercially canned green peas contains approximately 230 milligrams of sodium! One medium cucumber contains approximately 6 milligrams of sodium but one large dill pickle is estimated to hold 1,428 milligrams of sodium, or some 238 times what nature decreed! It just does not seem logical to this poor boy's critical faculties to believe that Providence intends us to be this heavy-handed with salt.

But this is only the tip of an iceberg. Canners know very well that salt stimulates the appetite. If the average American consumes 10 pounds annually (less than two of which are added at home) against the approximately one pound alleged by scientists to be a normal individual's requirement, there's small wonder high blood pressure kills so many good people in the prime of life. Insofar as raw vegetables are concerned, it is known that celery, beets, Swiss chard, dandelion greens, kale, spinach and turnips contain goodly amounts of "salts" but there is a world of nutritional difference between the assimilable organic salts contained naturally in these vegatables and the caustic salts utilized by the canning industry.

If I need additional salt in my food (which, remember, is the raw, unprocessed kind), I add powdered kelp (seaweed) which allegedly contains approximately twenty-one amino acids, twelve vitamins, sixty minerals and, of course, organic salts and iodine, all in a remarkable natural balance. Because of this, when not using kelp on raw vegetables, I not infrequently take six ten-grain kelp tablets before retiring. Each tablet contains 0.15 milligrams of organic iodine, or the Food and Drug Administration's recommended daily intake. Before ingesting iodine supplements in any form (for example, kelp or kelp tablets), be sure to have your doctor check your thyroid.

SUGGESTION 5: The average respiratory sufferer should avoid overeating. Overindulgence at the table puts too much strain on the digestive system, thus diverting energy away from the respiratory system. If the truth were fully known, as many people have probably dug their own graves with their spoons as have perished from all the pestilences, wars and accidents in history combined. It goes almost without saying that overindulgence is the root cause (in league with the wrong foods) of many human ailments.

SUGGESTION 6: If suffering an acute bronchial attack (with possible feverishness), it seems helpful to forgo solid foods for several days and consume instead a variety of healthful juices such as lemon or lime (somewhat diluted and honey-flavored), apple, cherry, orange, grapefruit, tangerine, pineapple, grape, cranberry, peach, carrot, apricot, or blackberry. Then one could try eating a variety of fresh whole fruits for a day or two before returning to a heavier, solid meal.

To loosen the attendant mucus deposits of such an attack, inhalation of steam from a hot shower bath or vaporizer may prove surprisingly helpful. This action could possibly be followed by pounding upon the chest with one's fingertips, shifting from one side to the other in the bed in an attempt to force the phlegm from the smaller bronchial tubes into the larger ones. Following this, one can lie face downward across the bed with the hands or forearms resting upon the floor on the other side (a narrow bed, of course, being best for shorter people). While the head is thus facing the floor, it may prove possible to cough up a quantity of loosened mucus into a special pan placed nearby for this purpose.

Hopefully, in the initial stages of the battle to combat a bronchial attack, a regular diet of healthful juices will promote a laxative condition and thus expedite the cleansing of the system. However, in order to receive sufficient nutrients, a good mineral-vitamin supplement of therapeutic strength can be taken along with the juice diet (and, for that matter, during the whole length of time one is rebuilding the body to conquer respiratory problems).

As can be seen, this is only a modified fast designed to momentarily curtail food intake without punishing a system already weakened by lengthy use of "foodless foods," respiratory drugs and, in some cases, the poison nicotine or alcoholic beverages in undue volume. Total fasting, of course, puts great strain upon the kidneys and liver, indeed the whole system, and should be carefully supervised by a physician. It is known that those functionally weak and malnourished could be harmed by fasting without a proper understanding of the subject. As for extended fasts, I cannot possibly believe they result in lasting benefits.

SUGGESTION 7: When one is generally exhausted, I've found a warm tub or shower bath prior to eating helps relax the body and aids the digestive processes. Moreover, always try to maintain a cheerful mood while eating. Experiments indicate the gall bladder is likely to produce excessive bile when one is unhappy, none when enraged, and the correct amount when of good cheer. Undoubtedly emotional distress can alter the gastric functions and thus inflame the mucous membranes. The respiratory sufferer should also delay exercising for at least an hour after eating because physical exertion may well interfere with digestion.

SUGGESTION 8: It is widely reported that allergy skin tests are to a considerable degree untrustworthy. Consequently, a patient may be placed on a less nourishing diet by his allergist because of a "positive reaction" to certain foods singled out by a skin test. Needless to say, someone can usually be found who is allergic to a specific food (or plant) that the overwhelming majority of the populace can abide without consequences.

Some raw foods (especially unwashed) may cause a reaction (albeit nonpermanent) of an allergic nature in some individuals. Among the more common offenders are various products derived from wheat or cow's milk, white potatoes, eggs, oranges, chocolate, shellfish, beef, onions, preservatives or food additives. It is also possible for allergic symptoms to spring from a drug reaction or an infection of some type. Well known nonfood culprits are plant pollens, trees such as ash, beech, birch, cedar, cypress, elder, elm, hickory, maple, oak, sycamore, and walnut. Other allergens are sundry chemicals, molds, various synthetic products, toiletries, old paper or books, dust in general, tobacco and the family pet.

How, then, in the absence of the much disowned skin test, are we to know what the offenders really are? This, admittedly, is no simple question, but early in my own crusade I realized that the human pulse may be a better "allergy barometer" than the skin test because the pulse not infrequently races when in close contact with an antagonistic force. Regarding this, I noted my pulse was rather often beating faster after "resting" in bed all night than it was before retiring and it seemed logical to assume this phenomenon was either triggered by something I had eaten before going to bed or was due to a nearby object to which I was allergic. I deduced that I was allergic to the mattress upon which I slept to some degree, so I was pleased to observe a certain drop in my morning pulse rate just before arising *after* I had covered my mattress with several additional sheets and thus blocked off some of the dust that naturally accumulates in mattresses, pillows, curtains, rugs, and so on.

I also observed that the more vital my health became the less my pulse raced and that I was in gradual stages increasing my ability to withstand allergenic forces whatever the source. After my respiratory allergies came under comfortable control, I learned that several physicians were utilizing scientific pulse testing techniques to determine which foods or "inhalants" caused a patient to undergo allergic symptoms and that the systematic restriction or elimination of the "antagonisms" brought about some rather astonishing improvements. In this connection, a patient was taught to record his pulse rate before arising, at the beginning of each of his three main meals, three times after each meal at thirty-minute intervals, and just before retiring at night. This totals fourteen pulse counts per day. (Pulse rates are timed for a full sixty seconds in order to get an accurate tally.) A record is also kept of the food(s) consumed for some five to ten days in order to establish a good trend.

According to the available research, one can (apart from foods) also use the pulse test to determine if he is allergic to house dust, cigarettes, medicines, fabrics, alcohol, cosmetics, etc., and can usually establish his minimum and maximum pulse rates within a few days. A variation of not more than two pulse beats per minute (between an individual's *daily maximum* readings) is to be hoped for after a substitution of nonallergenic food(s) for the offending one(s).

The maximum *normal daily* pulse *range* (or difference between counts) is reported to be sixteen beats. A count of eighty-four is considered the *maximum normal nonallergenic count* in an adult or child and the *normal* pulse is reported to be unaffected by *ordinary* activity or by nonallergenic food(s). An initial *allergenic pulse* may range from sixty-six to one hundred or more beats per minute. Upon removal of an allergenic food or substance the count may drop to a normal range of sixty-two to seventy-four, sixty-eight to eighty, fifty-two to sixty-six, forty-six to sixty-one, etc., per minute.

Of course, the pulse count can be sabotaged by drugs, an abnormally bulky meal, strenuous physical activity, or a body infection (such as the common cold). While it is possible to have a *normal* pulse rate of eighty or even more, any reading in excess of eighty-four is considered an allergenic one except as just noted. (Remember, it is best to take pulse readings calmly.)

It is alleged that, under *ordinary* conditions, a pulse beat six counts over an individual's *own* established *maximum normal rate* (which, as indicated, varies from person to person) could well be due to something inhaled (house dust, cigarette smoke, menthol in nose drops, perfumes or toiletries, soap powders, paint fumes, sundry chemicals or sprays, gasoline, ragweed, to name just a few) rather than a food allergy. If, then, a regularly eaten food does not accelerate an individual's pulse at least six beats above his carefully established maximum normal rate, the food is probably *not* allergenic.

Strangely enough, an individual with good resistance to the common cold reportedly manifests little or no allergic reactions to common foods although he may be adversely affected by a number of inhaled substances. Smoking tobacco is a notorious culprit and a pulse-taker under the sway of tobacco is specifically told to abandon this poisonous weed during the tests since 75 percent of the population has been deemed allergic to nicotine.

Although this is only a very brief summary of the pulse-test system of detecting allergy-causing foods or inhalants, anyone desiring to delve into this study at length should read *The Pulse Test* by Arthur F. Coca, M.D. (Arco Publishing Company, Inc., New York, N.Y.). However, if some item such as tobacco, egg, wheat, cow's milk, shellfish, sugar, walnuts, barbecue, sausage, coffee, or tea regularly causes a rapid rise of the pulse within a few minutes after consumption, one does not need to read Dr. Coca's book to suspect that the food involved should at least be avoided for the time being.

Of course great care should be exercised not to abandon a guiltless food of high value in the search for the real culprit(s), but if one suffers a consistent reaction such as hives, canker sores, indigestion, irritability, nausea, swellings or itchings, dizziness, stomach cramps, high blood pressure, fatigue, migraine, ordinary headaches, chest pains, neuralgia, colitis, constipation, diarrhea, or respiratory problems over a considerable span of time after eating some particular food(s), it appears the better part of wisdom to curtail or eliminate the offender(s).

Moreover, bear in mind that the pulse can be abnormally elevated by *ordinary* forces of the moment such as extreme temperatures, emotional tension, talking to someone shortly before or during a pulse test, not to mention less ordinary factors such as a coughing seizure, shortness of breath, fever, gluttony, overwork, or medicines. The *average* resting pulse count while seated is reportedly seventy-two to seventy-six beats per minute for men, seventy-five to eighty for women, eighty-two to eighty-nine for girls, and eighty to eighty-four for boys.

In any case, an elevated resting pulse rate is not an efficient one and, in general, the lower the reading the better. Interestingly, the mortality rate for adults is reported to be four times greater among those with resting pulse rates over ninety-two than for those with readings under sixty-seven beats a minute. As the pulse rate diminishes, the heart accordingly labors less strenuously and the body's oxygen supply is increased. This fact has important implications for the respiratory sufferer and demonstrates the need to develop a vital physical fitness plan in conjunction with a vital food program!

SUGGESTION 9: Chew your meals slowly and completely. This is an exceedingly important step in a most complicated digestive operation. And the less strain you put on your digestive system, the more effectively it will work—and this means your respiratory system will also operate more easily.

SUGGESTION 10: Study food value charts and learn the vitamin-mineral contents of foods so that you can design for yourself the most beneficial diet possible. Many of the food values given in such charts represent canned or processed foods fully imbued with salt, white sugar, and other detrimental ingredients. One can only imagine how much greater the nutritional worth must have been in many foods, vegetables in particular, *before* they reached the canneries. Heat destroys or modifies many natural elements, especially enzymes so essential to the digestive process.

Fortunately many fruits, nuts, and vegetables are evaluated in their raw state. While studying the charts, one may be astonished by the outstandingly high level of Vitamin A found in dandelion greens, a valuable plant that grows wild over most of the countryside and is free for the taking.

While I have seen no data on rose hips (the seed pods of roses gathered after the petals have fallen off), approximately four of them are said to contain as much Vitamin C as a medium-sized orange (90 milligrams). There are some wild roses in my area and I frequently eat the rose hips *whole*, in season, while still tender, before the outside cover becomes leathery. In this way I consume a wide range of nutrients including Vitamin E, along with the Vitamin C. However, the Vitamin C-laden seeds inside the rose hip pods can be separated and dried. Ground to a powder and sprinkled on salads, this is a wonderful source of Vitamin C. One should *not* attempt to chew the rose hips after the hardening process has set in, because there is no humor involved in having a tooth cracked during the effort!

Studying the food-composition charts will no doubt cause the respiratory sufferer to shun radical diets lacking in the proper mineral-vitamin balance. Regarding this, disciples of the Zen macrobiotic diet in its most zealous form have reportedly expired from consuming naught save water and brown rice for an extended period of time. While brown rice is certainly valuable consumed *with other foods*, it is woefully lacking in B2, folic acid, and calcium, and contains absolutely zero in the way of Vitamins A and C.

Despite the invaluable aid of food-composition charts in formulating a vital food program, they can only go so far and cannot educate us to the fact that thyme in excess can trigger internal upsets; that mango peelings may be toxic; that excessive amounts of rosemary can result in death if taken internally; that too much nutmeg can produce serious side effects; that the presence of oxalic acid (toxic in undue volume) in spinach, rhubarb, Swiss chard and beet greens can apparently interfere with the body's calcium absorption; that potato sprouts (eyes) or any green part of the peeling should definitely not be consumed because of the poison solanine contained therein; that apple or pear seeds contain cyanide (as do the pits of apricots, peaches, nectarines, plums or cherries); that honey derived from the toxic nectars of rhododendron, oleander, mountain laurel, azalea, or yellow jessamine (mercifully rare in the marketplace) should *not* be consumed; that the preservative waxes on supermarket fruits and vegetables may cause allergic reactions in some individuals; or that acute illness has resulted from consuming an edible mushroom called inky cap in combination with alcoholic beverages.

These suggestions should prove of benefit in the gradual improvement, control, or cure of a number of diverse human ailments in addition to the allergic symptoms of asthma, bronchitis, hay fever, rhinitis, conjunctivitis, sinusitis and hopefully emphysema. Of course, a vital food program travels hand in hand with the proper rest, exercise, fresh air (if available!), sunshine, recreation, vitamin-mineral therapy, herbal knowledge, emotional balance, and self-discipline if the maximum victory is to be had!

Other points to be considered in formulating a vital food program follow.

FOOD FOR THOUGHT: Reportedly, allergies to a food do not develop if the food is thoroughly digested. Although indigestion plagued me fearfully prior to my development of a vital food program, a skin test given me by an allergist indicated that I was allergic to just about every thing on earth *except* food! Perhaps, at that time, cigarette smoke, animal dander, dust, mildew, pollens, and so on *were* responsible for my inability to digest my food (as well as my worsening respiratory ills) but, in retrospect, I believe my rather abominable eating habits played an important role in causing my various allergies.

Whatever the truth, I believed my allergist knew his business since he had M.D. affixed to his name and the size of my bill led me to suspect that he must, indeed, be a man of exceptional understanding if not genius. Thank God I had the hindsight to decline the series of desensitization shots he recommended since, by now, there is a better than even chance my bronchial ailments would have degenerated into emphysema. None of this is said with rancor inasmuch as most allergists are doing their best and sick people are by no means easy to deal with. After all, a little "progress" may have been made in allergy testing because in the early days thereof it was not uncommon to present sufferers with lists of forbidden items in excess of 400!

FOOD FOR THOUGHT: Ponder well the old Chinese proverb that declares "Man who drinks medicine but eats badly wastes doctors' knowledge."

FOOD FOR THOUGHT: Some five centuries prior to the advent of Christ, the Greek physician Hippocrates informed his students "Thy food shall be thy remedy." With cancer rampant in the land—not to speak of a multitude of other grave ailments—only a small percentage of a huge outlay of money appropriated to combat cancer has been spent to *prevent* this curse through proper diet or mineral-vitamin therapy. The same logic applies for respiratory allergies as well. It is high time the laws of nature took some priority over the wonder-drug craze abroad in the land.

FOOD FOR THOUGHT: Since the general population has been programmed from birth to consume cooked food, the taste buds have accordingly been perverted, modified or enfeebled to such a degree that the average person will have to experience gradually the altogether superior taste of unsalted, unprocessed and uncooked foods in the natural state.

It is, of course, almost impossible to live in a completely "natural" way in today's world but I usually manage to consume raw foods for my first two meals. My third (evening) meal may be partially cooked or processed since I rather frequently consume several slices of whole-grain bread (without preservatives), soured milk products in small amounts (buttermilk, cottage cheese, or yogurt), in order to gain sufficient calcium and Vitamin B12, a few eggs, or tuna fish (the dietetic or low-sodium canned type).

FOOD FOR THOUGHT: Proceed slowly and cautiously. In designing a vital food program, it may not be wise to abolish everything that seems (at the time) to be mucus-forming as this may well deprive an already weakened system of essential elements and thus do more damage in the long run than good. The temperate and gradual control of asthma, bronchitis, and hay fever has advantages that total "crash programs" do not.

As a general rule, one should *gradually* decrease prescribed or over-the-counter medicines because the system has become so utterly dependent upon them over a long period of time. In my own case, I felt it necessary to slowly decrease my respiratory medicines over a period of six months. Approximately six months after that I had (hopefully) my last asthma attack!

FOOD FOR THOUGHT: Many medicines, including the decongestants upon which respiratory sufferers depend so heavily, stubbornly remain in the system a good while after their use is discontinued. Aspirin is evidently guilty of this persistence and some asthmatics (as many as 20 percent, by one estimate) may be allergic to aspirin. Aspirin has long been accused of contributing to ulcers, internal bleedings, ear noises, among other problems. This should cause us to ponder well the thought that not infrequently our best medicine is the food we eat!

FOOD FOR THOUGHT: It is believed that the adrenal and pituitary glands—which produce antihistamine secretions under normal conditions—are exhausted by some of the allegedly safe drugs on the market. Moreover, drugs are known to have destructive effects upon the body's mineral-vitamin-enzyme storehouse at the same time they are masking or suppressing respiratory conditions and killing germs.

While undoubtedly there are times when one should

not hesitate to take a particular drug to immobilize a bad infection or certain dangerous germs, one should at the same time try to build oneself up with vitamin-mineral supplements and to eat the proper foods. This should aid the body in mobilizing its own natural powers of recuperation which, all too often, are suppressed by the drugs prescribed by physicians who ought to be recommending a vital food program instead.

While I realize that a fairly large number of sufferers would not embrace *any* plan designed to restore the body's ability to repair itself, the medical profession should throw a greater fear of God into more patients with respect to their abominable eating habits. It is easier, of course, to write a prescription for a drug, than to risk awakening them to the fact that a vital diet might well prolong their lives by many years (and play hell with hospital economics). This is not said with malevolent intent, but is based instead on my observations. Here again let it be emphasized that in no small degree food is our best medicine because WE ARE WHAT WE EAT. Even people with inborn weaknesses or defects have been known to enjoy considerable improvements through proper exercise, sun, fresh air, mineral-vitamin therapy, and *living* foods!

FOOD FOR THOUGHT: Remember that the more longstanding and acute the respiratory complaint, the slower the improvement is apt to be. But remember also that the orthodox medical profession with its vested interest has an exceedingly poor track record in the control, much less cure, of respiratory malfunctions. The use of such potent drugs as Isuprel or Isoproterenol and cortisone in its several erratic forms can prove worse than the original complaint. What lasting good is there in relieving an asthma attack if a cortisone drug *interacts* with an aerosol spray asthma medication such as Isuprel, Norisodrine or Duo-Medihaler already in the system and produces the same sort of fatal heart rhythms in humans as those reportedly induced in laboratory animals? This is said not to frighten the asthmatic sufferer but rather to spur the reader into action dietwise!

FOOD FOR THOUGHT: Notwithstanding the marvels of modern food technology, mankind can never equal or improve upon what nature has supplied for the proper maintenance of the human body. In a very real sense, there is no known way we can keep on subtracting and end up having as much as we started with. From here on, I hope that the reader will pay as much attention to the quality of food he puts in his body as the fuel he uses in his automobile.

FOOD FOR THOUGHT: In order to obtain the right kinds of food in this pollution-hazed society, I would suggest that those with sufficient land plant an organic garden. Not only can this prove a praiseworthy hobby and perhaps an economic godsend, but the fresh produce harvested should be superior to virtually anything purchased from the supermarkets at the going rate.

FOOD FOR THOUGHT: The blessings are manifold for those who weary not in welldoing but we must keep our wits about us at all times and the respiratory sufferer should ponder well the old prayer: God grant me the serenity to accept the things I cannot change; the courage to change the things I can; and the wisdom to know the difference.

CHAPTER III

HONEY—THE NECTAR OF THE GODS

Besides being a natural substitute for sugar, honey has many other advantages that make it of great value to respiratory sufferers. I have found it invaluable in my encounters with bronchial congestion and, to a great extent, with my old adversary hay fever.

Amazingly, honey is reputed to be 99 percent pre-digested. According to a number of studies, it enters the blood stream in under half an hour. Because of its sedative properties, honey calms or relaxes the entire respiratory system. I have found that several dolomite or bone meal tablets in a warm glass of buttermilk with several teaspoons of honey bring about more restful sleep than anything sold in a drug store. Doctors of an earlier era often recommended a tablespoon or two of honey by itself as a sleep-inducer, or had the patients mix several tablespoonfuls with hot milk, water or lemon juice just before retiring.

Severe asthmatic spasms have been relieved for some by ingesting one teaspoonful of honey every quarter hour. Several teaspoons of althaea or marsh mallow roots (Althaea officinalis) boiled in honey and water have also been used for bronchial wheezings, coughs, shortness of breath, hoarseness and restlessness. Respiratory sufferers with insomnia might try, just before bedtime, squeezing one orange and one lemon (or lime) into hot water, adding several tablespoons of honey, and slowly drinking this natural nervine mixture. To safely relax the system prior to retiring at night, an asthmatic might alternatively try dropping one full teaspoon of either balm (lemon or sweet), catnip, or skullcap into a cup of water *after* it has reached the boiling point. Let this steep for about half an hour (covered with a lid to retain all the vital elements), strain and flavor with several teaspoonfuls of honey before drinking. Some may wish to rewarm this herbal tea after allowing it to steep, but I achieved successful results without doing so. (The three herbs mentioned have, in due course, a safe antispasmodic effect on congested bronchial tubes in addition to calming the average nervous system.)

I soon realized that the linings of the digestive tract were not irritated by honey and that goodly amounts of it (together with my largely raw food regimen) did not cause a gain in weight despite the fact that an average tablespoonful contained sixty-four calories. And for quick energy, honey is virtually unsurpassed.

Depending upon its source, raw honey contains in varying degrees the digestive enzymes diastase, inulase, invertase, lipase, oxidase, peroxidase; vital amino acids used in protein synthesis so important in tissue repair; other valuable acids such as acetic, butyric, citric, cluconic, formic, lactic, malic, pyroglutamic, succinic, and tartaric; antiseptic properties that inhibit the growth of microorganisms; a bactericidal substance known as inhibine; sugar alcohols; ester compounds; sundry pigments; royal jelly; beeswax; desensitized pollens; and fifteen different natural sugars including glucose. (The body's digestive juices eventually convert all sugars and starches into glucose, also known as blood sugar.)

Interestingly, all asthmatics reportedly have low blood sugar and have allegedly received relief from glucose shots that raised their blood sugar level. Asthma attacks of the most fearful kind frequently occur in the early hours of the morning when the level of blood sugar dips to the lowest point. (This is another reason to take some honey at bedtime—to keep the blood sugar level high throughout the night.) Strangely enough, asthma is virtually unknown among diabetics whose blood sugar levels are very high, and in instances where asthmatics became diabetics their asthma reportedly ceased. Moreover, experiments indicate that asthmatics are adversely affected by consumption of salt in undue volume whereas salt reportedly lessens the insulin needs of diabetics.

One wonders how many people would have become diabetic if their sugar supply had been derived from fresh fruits and honey. At one time, diabetics were said to have been successfully treated by homeopathic physicians with honey and improved diets. Observers report that diabetes is not common in primitive societies that consume honey in place of white sugar. It is also interesting that in 1929, one of the discoverers of insulin, Sir Frederick Banting, declared, "In the United States, the incidence of diabetes has increased proportionately with the per capita consumption of cane sugar. In the heating and recrystallization of the natural cane sugar, something is altered which leaves the refined product a dangerous foodstuff." This should make us pause to consider the virtues of honey, one of nature's most magnificent gifts.

While the darker varieties of honey have several times more food value than the lighter ones, the vitamin-mineral content of honey is generally measured in micrograms instead of milligrams. Although many foods outrank this marvelously compounded, predigested, enzyme-packed nectar of the gods in vitamin-mineral content, their assimilability cannot compare with that of honey.

It should be noted here that the beautiful "homogenized" appearance of most honey sold in the supermarkets is due to subjecting it to high temperatures in order to prevent it from hardening or looking cloudy in the bottles. The fact that 35 percent of the food value may be destroyed in the process becomes secondary to commercial considerations. Realizing this, I purchase uncooked honey from the health center in five-pound containers. Of course, if honey becomes hardened from being stored, it can be slowly warmed until a liquid state is reached again.

The *hygroscopic* power of honey—the natural ability to readily attract or hold moisture—makes it impossible for germs or microorganisms to live in it! This bactericidal power holds promise for the control of respiratory ailments. Properly capped (to prevent moisture intake), honey has the ability to remain unspoiled for phenomenal periods of time. Egyptologists have claimed that honey taken from tombs of the Pharaohs of ancient Egypt was still edible without any adverse side effects. (Indeed, honey may be the true wonder substance of all time. It has historically been used to prevent bed-wetting in children because of its moisture-holding properties. And it is also claimed that cancer is not very often met with in beekeepers who eat their own product regularly.)

But honey is not the only beneficial substance produced by bees. Royal jelly is a rare substance secreted by the glands of worker bees. It is fed to new colony members for three days after hatching. Following this, however, royal jelly is the exclusive diet of the exceedingly vibrant queen bee who may, astonishingly, live seventy times as long as the undersized workers and lay twice her own bulk in eggs daily. For humans, apart from its ability to lessen arthritic woes, royal jelly is praised as an aid in the control of respiratory afflictions because it is apparently uncommonly rich in the B-complex vitamins biotin and pantothenic acid, with a lesser quantity of pyridoxine.

While pollen is both a vital part of honey and, according to allergists, the enemy in many cases (particularly during ragweed season), there appears to be no evidence that the regular use of pollen is anything less than beneficial. It's my theory that God has not *told* the bees that pollen is the enemy but, not knowing this, they have systematically proceeded to desensitize it in transforming it into honey. After all, are they not the earth's greatest chemists?

Unprocessed honey contains greater amounts of pollen than industry-filtered honey. It is claimed that primitive tribes who eat pollen as a way of life are remarkably free of hay fever, asthma, bronchitis or respiratory complaints. If true, this amounts to a simple oral consumption of the various pollens to which one might, in a technological society, be strongly allergic and, in consequence, receive desensitization injections from an overeducated allergist. Of course, there is more to the control of respiratory allergies than eating pollen alone. But I believe that after more study and testing, it will be found that pollen tablets, along with other effective aids, can be beneficial to many asthmatics. Undoubtedly, pollen is one very valuable ingredient in the overall construction of the miracle food we call honey.

Although I had always been vaguely aware of honey as a natural sweetener, it was my brother Douglas who first suggested that the regular eating of raw (locally found) honey and the chewing of honeycomb might bring about the following advantageous results: (1) a soothing effect upon the bronchial tubes and mucous membranes of the nasal passages during an asthma, bronchitis or hay fever attack; (2) relief to itching eyes so common to the hay fever victim; (3) a drying up of the watery condition of both the eyes and nasal passages; and (4) an all-around good effect upon the digestive processes, body chemistry and vital organs (aside from those of the respiratory system).

Being desperate, I did not question my brother's claims as to the possible therapeutic values of honey. Instead, in February, 1973, I began taking honey and honeycomb seriously. Sometimes I took several teaspoons of raw honey alone and evaluated the results carefully. After what appeared to be a reasonable period of time, I chewed a good sized chunk of honey-filled comb for thirty or forty minutes until almost nothing remained of it. Then I again took several teaspoons of the honey and promptly followed this action with a lengthy honeycomb-chewing session.

After a few days of experimentation, I sensed that relief from the miseries of hay fever and bronchial congestion was at hand. So I began chewing honeycomb three or four times daily after taking the liquid honey. While I appreciated the soothing effect of the treatment on my congested lower respiratory system, I was particularly grateful for the partial abatement of watery discharges (from my eyes and nasal passages) and especially for the reduction in itching (and inflammation) of my eyes.

Later still I found that itching, watery or inflamed eyes seemed to respond just as well to either (1) a little extra Vitamin A, though not in toxic quantities; (2) ingestion of a twenty-five-milligram riboflavin (B2) tablet in addition to the ten milligrams already received from my basic multivitamin-mineral capsule formula taken daily (which is described in a coming chapter); or (3) an increase in the intake of Vitamin C which is widely declared to be a lot safer than the antihistamine or decongestant drugs on the market. A still better method is herbal smoking (discussed in a later chapter). This should be considered if *rapid* relief is sought on occasion (*without sacrificing the gradual internal revitalization of the body* achievable through proper diet, elimination of body wastes, honey consumption, vitamin-mineral therapy, and exercise).

As for the use of Vitamin C, one well-known study states it is "essentially nontoxic" but that "5,000-10,000 milligrams daily over a prolonged period may have side effects in some persons."[1] I do not believe in ingesting too much of anything and rarely take more than three

---

[1] John D. Kirschmann, *Nutrition Almanac* (New York: McGraw-Hill, 1975), p. 44.

thousand milligrams of Vitamin C in a day's time, but I do find the controversial views of Dr. Linus Pauling on the matter of Vitamin C of interest. In the January, 1977, issue of *The Body Forum*, Pauling is quoted as declaring, "All current cold medications can affect only the symptoms of a cold and cannot stop a cold. Many of these medications are toxic in large doses. Vitamin C has never been shown to be toxic even in doses as large as a quarter of a pound." I assume Dr. Pauling was not actually advising here the use of Vitamin C for respiratory disorders in this outrageous quantity but was trying to emphasize the safety of the vitamin.

As for himself, Pauling claims to ingest ten thousand milligrams daily of Vitamin C, one thousand-two hundred units of Vitamin E and a multivitamin tablet which provides four thousand units of Vitamin A. He is further quoted in *The Body Forum* as saying, "Today cold medicines carry the warning KEEP THIS MEDICINE OUT OF REACH OF CHILDREN. I think they should say: KEEP THIS MEDICINE OUT OF REACH OF EVERYBODY! USE ASCORBIC ACID INSTEAD! Vitamin C is completely nontoxic, unlike the cold drugs, all of which are toxic, and some of which may cause serious side effects."

I not infrequently chew a five-hundred-milligram Vitamin C tablet completely if confronted with any degree of hay fever and modify the bittersweet flavor with several teaspoonfuls of organic honey without water (although I may later rinse my mouth out somewhat as possible dental protection).

While it may appear that I am advocating the complete nonuse of drugs, I have no doubt that there are instances where a properly diagnosed ailment may require a specific medicine; however, it does not appear that drugs as we know them actually "cure" disease and, on the whole, there *must* surely be a better way—particularly in the matter of *forestallment* programs. An ounce of prevention may actually be worth a pound of cure, just as the old adage says! I believe that the faithful use of honey is only one of nature's gifts that, if properly used, can gradually bring about the best medical treatment or remedy.

If one suffers from seasonal hay fever or sinus attacks, he may possibly build up some immunity by chewing honeycomb on a regular basis *several months* in advance of the "season" and also crutail the toxic drugs he would ordinarily consume. And after consultation with his doctor, he may also wish to take Vitamin C, eat honey itself regularly, and ingest pollen tablets as a further preventive measure.

I know of no evidence that the honeycomb (after chewing) is harmful. However, the residue must be the purest form of wax and I feel it *surely best* to discard the surplus, although a number of people swallow honeycomb at the breakfast table as a matter of course, claiming no ill effects at all. Honeycomb is honey in its rawest form and only God knows what beeswax is composed of. Some people call the pollen-loaded and marvelously sealed combs "honeycaps," and the reader interested in honeycomb therapy should seek out a local beekeeper who can quote him a fair price on several pounds of partially moist "cappings" sliced from the honeycombs or even entire blocks of comb wax with enough honey remaining to impart moisture and thus prevent drying out. When my hay fever was in the chronic stages, I had several pounds of honeycomb stored in the refrigerator at all times. (I purchased a very fine sourwood variety from Mr. D. A. Ratley of Red Springs, North Carolina. He can also astound one with his knowledge of bees.)

The darker varieties of honey, it is reported, have greater alkaline values than the lighter types. The chewing of honeycomb is said to aid inflamed sinus cavities by changing the balance of urine from alkaline to acid. On the other hand, honey is widely praised for its ability to decrease digestive disturbances attributable to excess acidity. One should not be surprised at anything honey does. By regulating the thyroid glands, iodine-rich seaweed is said to help those who are underweight *as well as* those who are overweight. So perhaps honey has the somewhat similar ability to regulate the body's alkaline-acid chemistry.

During some asthmatic seizures (or where possible before they increased in intensity) I also received bronchial relief from combining raw honey with pure Mazola (low in saturated fats) corn oil and swallowing three or four tablespoons of the mixture. This seems to have a coating action that relaxes the bronchial tubes and I obtained some relief from the coughing, wheezing, choking, quickened pulse, digestive tract turmoil, and shallowness of breath that are so much a part of the seizures. I was later told that doctors in the past (comparatively uneducated, of course, in the use of high velocity drugs) would often give an asthmatic child two tablespoons of pure olive oil followed promptly by several teaspoons (or tablespoons if possible) of warm honey to make the dose more palatable. If this combination was given before bedtime the child usually slept throughout the night.

I have read that one should take an additional one hundred International Units of Vitamin E daily for every tablespoonful of vegetable oil consumed in excess of two. I was not able to accurately evaluate this theory since my consumption of Vitamin E was simultaneously so great (varying from eight hundred to twelve hundred International Units daily depending on the stresses upon me) and, as near as I can determine, my corn oil ingestions did not interfere with the favorable circulatory actions of Vitamin E one way or another. This may have been due to the fact that my system was well saturated with Vitamin E on a daily basis as noted in chapter 1. If you decide to try taking corn oil and honey, it might be wise to increase your intake of Vitamin E as well.

I also believe that two teaspoons of honey mixed with two teaspoons of *pure*, full strength (5.5 percent acidity) apple cider "medicinal" vinegar in a glass of water (taken two or three times daily) will aid the average person suffering from respiratory ailments. This is an old arthritis remedy and only vinegar made from the pure apple *juice* should be used. Apple cider vinegar in the small amounts indicated will apparently not thin the blood dangerously and anyway people often use considerably more than this on their salads. In any case, apple cider vinegar is a health food in its own right and has often been used with honey on a regular basis for curbing bad "nerves," migraine headaches, intestinal disorders, dizziness, insomnia, and stomach troubles, in addition to allegedly aiding hay fever, asthma, bronchitis, and the gout. From my own experience, I feel that apple cider vinegar and honey used together may aid in lessening the pulse rate.

Some people claim they are able to alleviate a hay fever attack by merely ingesting two or three teaspoons of honey at the outset and following this with additional honey at appropriate times thereafter. Sneezing fits are also allegedly halted for some by eating as few as two cloves, while drinking clove tea reportedly stops nausea.

Honey and diluted lemon juice (or apple cider vinegar) have long been used as gargles to treat colds, relieve coughs, and alleviate sore throats. When gargled, there appears to be no particular harm in swallowing the mixture. While most people would probably prefer to dilute the lemon juice, it is said to be superior when used undiluted.

The health-giving properties of honey are regarded by many as having no equal in the history of medicine. It has its advocates for treating third-degree burns, weak hearts, high blood pressure (with lemon juice added), skin ailments of numerous kinds (including deep flesh wounds), gangrenous feet or legs (when an operation might kill a very weak patient, completely covering the infected limb with organic honey is a last resort), fatigue, prostate troubles (pure pollen is used), and internal ulcers. Our sacred writings exalt honey's virtues and the ancient Egyptians glorified it on their monuments even going so far as to depict beekeepers subduing bees with smoke to render them manageable. In 1919, a rock painting said to date from 12,000 B.C. was discovered in a cave near Valencia, Spain, depicting "beekeepers" taking honey from a nest of obviously angry bees by use of a smoke-producing substance.

When we learn that it takes four pounds of nectar to make a pound of honey, which contains the essence of an estimated two million flowers, only then do we begin to realize the prize that is honey! Perhaps people began using white sugar because they thought it was more economical. As for real economic considerations, however, honey is an investment in good health.

CHAPTER IV

FORMULATING A DETOXIFICATION PROGRAM

In order to eliminate or control respiratory disorders, allergy sufferers must formulate their own detoxification program based on the safest methods possible. Those sufferers also afflicted with chronic constipation need all the ammunition they can get. Uneliminated waste materials gradually create a state of internal pollution and toxic poisons can thereby "overflow" from the intestines into the blood stream without the victims realizing that they are slowly being "self-poisoned" (known medically as autointoxication). Yet, surprisingly enough, few pople ever really think of this as their vital organs fail them little by little.

In due time, the respiratory sufferer should be well on his way to improved health after embracing the vital food program outlined in chapter 2, especially SUG-GESTIONS No. 1 (on the intake of *predominately* raw foods), No. 2 (on *comparatively moderate* protein intake), No. 3 (on the before or after mealtime intake of fresh juices and herbal teas), and No. 4 (on the elimination of white sugar and salt from the diet where possible). Thus also is war declared against a wide range of junk food, including the unnatural white bread, nonassimilable food additives, and untrustworthy starches (such as spaghetti and macaroni).

It must be remembered that while possibly mucus-forming in excess, starch (a carbohydrate) is valuable in the digestive process because enzymes break it down into various sugars which in turn produce energy. Staple foods with high starch content are potatoes, soybeans, rice, cereal grains, (wheat, rye, oats, etc.), and corn. Sunflower seeds, Brazil nuts, peanuts, almonds, cashews, hazelnuts, chestnuts, and pumpkin or sesame seeds are also starch sources and suppliers of energy as well as valuable nonmeat protein-packed foodstuffs. *Natural* starch is, indeed, vital.

It is widely held that one should not eat heavy meals if overly tense or fatigued. Also one should, for a time, either eat nothing solid or else very lightly when suffering from a fever (a frequent accompaniment to bronchitis). Fever is believed to be nature's way of telling the body it needs a rest.

In this connection the reader may consider SUGGES-TION No. 6 (chapter 2) which deals with the temporary use of fresh juices, along with a basic multivitamin-mineral capsule (containing B12 so lacking in juices). To this one may add extra Vitamin A (mucous membrane repair factor), Vitamin E (apparently a circulatory-oxygen improvement factor), Vitamin C (antihistamine factor), B2 (itching eyes factor), B6 (antihistamine factor), pantothenic acid (antihistamine factor in some instances), several bone meal tablets to supply calcium (involved in heart-nerve-muscle functions) and a little additional Vitamin D from a natural source to insure calcium absorption.

Stomach pains after a substantial meal are often believed to be a result of too much stomach acid. But sometimes when one takes drug store alkalizers, gas problems and even vomiting are experienced. This is because the victim is actually suffering from a *deficiency* of hydrochloric acid in his stomach. A doctor would then take the sufferer off alkalizer tablets because the patient needs *more* acid instead of *less*. However, products such as betaine or glutamic hydrochloric tablets, commonly found in health food stores, as well as papaya or pineapple-derived enzyme tablets also relieve stomach problems by restoring the acid balance and aiding in the digestion of protein. Lemon or apple juices often aid digestive processes too. Of course, it is wise in cases of persistent indigestion (along with clay-colored evacuations and intestinal gas) to consult a physician to make certain the ailment is not caused by diseases of the gall bladder, pancreas or liver.

Some advocates of natural foods believe that digestive disorders stemming from stomach ulcers can be relieved by the alkalizing actions of raw cabbage juice (up to six four-ounce glasses a day), or the juice of raw white potatoes, or those same potatoes cooked to an utter pulp and thoroughly mashed. (See Bibliography for books dealing with natural remedies.) Digestive upsets can also be minimized by *completely* chewing foods in a relaxed environment. For some adults who suffer digestive disturbances from drinking commercial sweet milk, the remedy may be to switch to fermented lactic acid products such as buttermilk, cottage cheese and yogurt. Digestive tumult is also frequently caused by the poison nicotine, as well as by refined, superbly packaged, artificially colored, low-fiber, deceitfully ballyhooed junk food.

The most important detoxification weapon in overcoming chronic constipation is the regular consumption of *raw fruits, vegetables and juices* (as a water source) until a normal, regular, evacuation pattern is established. One can, however, obtain valuable results from regularly consuming *dried* fruits such as prunes, figs, dates, apricots, peaches, apples, or raisins. Likewise, dried prunes or figs can be covered with honey (also a mild laxative) and lemon juice and then soaked in a container of hot water overnight. The liquid should be consumed before breakfast the following morning. The prunes or figs may also be eaten for breakfast along with fresh fruits, vegetables and unsalted, nutritious, protein-laden sunflower seeds, almonds or peanuts.

Fortunately, almost any variety of fresh fruit in goodly quantity has the tendency to encourage a laxative condition. I have found, however, that wild blackberries (several local species), eaten in abundance, are a little clodpating, although valuable as a wild food in moderation. (The roots and leaves of wild blackberries have been used as a home remedy since early times to control diarrhea and perhaps some of this power has found its way into the berries!) Also, anyone with an overacid condition should avoid plums, gooseberries, and cranberries (or even prunes). There are also reports that peanuts, walnuts and Brazil nuts may be acid-forming on occasion. However, these can be valuable foods eaten in *proper* amounts under *normal* conditions.

Eating a large amount of bran in cereals or breads may actually retard proper evacuation at times whereas the addition of two teaspoons of bran to the diet three times daily is considered a roughage source of definite value in preventing constipation.

Prompt obedience to the call of nature is important in conquering constipation woes but those with hemorrhoids, heart problems, or other conditions must avoid straining at the stool. I cannot resist the conviction a twice daily laxative condition (without straining) is devoutly to be hoped for despite a rather frequently voiced medical opinion that "every soul has his time" and that waiting three days for action is "normal." Whatever the truth, one should establish a *regular* toilet schedule and abide by it. Failure to do this can foster dependence upon commercial laxatives, many of which are unsafe, or mineral oils that may interfere with one's normal absorption of Vitamins A, D and E in addition to other important nutrients.

The Palomar Mountain Observatory telescope might be helpful in reading the undersized instructions on some of the attractively packaged laxative formulas but, I hope, most laxative addicts know these potions should be avoided in cases of nausea, vomiting or other signs of appendicitis. (Moreover, pregnant women should *not* take laxatives of any kind.)

Apart from proper eating habits, the use of *warm water enemas* may be one of the best detoxification weapons available for some respiratory sufferers. About a quart of warm water is usually allowed to gradually enter the colon from a bag hanging on the wall a foot or two above one's self. If there is an urge to evacuate too rapidly after the warm water enters the body, one can control the flow rate by use of a clamp on the rubber tube coming from the water bag. By shutting the water off or on, the hardened materials in the colon are given several minutes to loosen or dissolve before one reaches the stool to complete the evacuation process.

If, upon reading thus far, anyone is interested in taking an enema, lie on the left side upon the floor with the knee of one's right leg bent toward the chest so the water can better flow into the body with, perhaps, a piece of plastic material underneath to catch any discharge that occurs before leaping up (hopefully) to locate the stool. The enema tip should be lubricated with olive oil before insertion to make entry easier and, according to authorities, insertion should be about three inches and NEVER in excess of four. Again, let there be no straining while attending stool! Also, the beginner who is not acquainted with this old-fashioned way of purging the body of toxic waste may find it helpful to solicit the advice of a veteran in the business or initially test one of the disposable enema outfits—in accordance with directions—commonly sold in corner pharmacies.

I believe my vitamin-mineral program (to be discussed later) is also of value in the overall detoxification of the mucus-clogged system. And do not be surprised to learn that health food stores sell much blackstrap molasses for drinking regularly with honey to promote regularity. I believe this natural aid to elimination is also worthy of consideration.

For some people, and I am one of them, Kelp is an effective laxative. I take six ten-grain kelp tablets before retiring at night and have good results upon arising next day. This intake is six times the FDA's recommended consumption, although one famed nutritionist advocates taking fifteen to twenty-five kelp tablets daily. I personally would *not* consume this volume even though kelp is a natural iodine source.

Edible kelp (*Alaria esculenta*), found from Massachusetts northward, has enjoyed some popularity as a foodstuff and is said to have a sweet taste. In addition to its value in combating goiter, much has been written with regard to kelp's use for asthma, anemia, rickets, stomach disorders, headaches, eczema, nervousness, prostate troubles, indigestion, high blood pressure, female ailments, intestinal autotoxemia (self-poisoning) and constipation. It is also said to be of value in the control of bronchitis, colds, coughs, slow-healing wounds and rheumatism. In bygone days it was used for problems of the liver, gall bladder, pancreas, bile duct, and kidneys.

A number of assimilable minerals and vitamins are found in kelp and one ten-grain tablet contains two milligrams of natural iron. As is well known, a deficiency of iron results in anemia, skin paleness, sluggishness and constipation. If you are interested in trying kelp for any reason, check with your doctor first. Be sure to ask him how taking kelp would affect your thyroid.

Fenugreek (*Trigonella foenumgaecumgraecum*) may be of gradual benefit to some people. It has been used since the Pharaos for bronchitis, tuberculosis, fevers, colds, sore throats (gargled), general swellings, mucous membrane inflammations, and to "cool" the bowels. Along with iron and lecithin, it contains mucilage (which lubricates the intestines without irritation and provides bulk) thus aiding elimination. When the seeds are made into tea, the bitter taste can be disguised with honey. Fenugreek is also sold in tablet form by some health centers.

Slippery elm tablets (sold primarily as throat lozenges), while not used for constipation, do have diuretic properties. They are also soothing to the mucous membranes in much the same manner as fenugreek if consumed regularly. Slippery elm (*Ulmus fulva*) can be purchased in several forms. The inner bark seems to have a long medicinal history for "bronchitis" but is scarcely mentioned as a "specific" in fighting asthma. Slippery elm is ranked by herbalists as demulcent, emollient, expectorant and nutritive, as well as diuretic. The inner bark is also considered of value for diarrhea or dysentery and is said to be especially good for inflammations of the kidneys, stomach and bowels.

In the early days of my detoxification program I continued to suffer from acidity, indigestion, gas, and heartburn but I found that chewing a teaspoon or two of anise seeds (*Pimpinella anisum*) was the best neutralizing method available. It was also a welcome substitute for the commercial antacids I formerly depended on with their contents of aspirin (for its pain-killing ability evidently), sodium bicarbonate (definitely not recommended for anyone on a low-salt diet), calcium carbonate (which, after initially lessening acidity, stimulates the stomach to produce excess acidity and howl for *more* calcium carbonate), and aluminum hydroxide (which, in undue strength, reportedly produces constipation).

Although anise seeds belong to the carrot family, their taste resembles that of licorice to which they bear no botanical kinship whatever. In addition to their aromatic, digestive, gas-expelling, and stomach-strengthening properties, anise seeds have certain expectorant and antispasmodic abilities. They are used commercially to lessen the griping action of purgative-strength laxatives. Doctors in earlier times seem to have used anise seed tea to combat the dry coughs of bronchitis where expectoration comes with difficulty. I have also received bronchial relief by smoking anise seeds in a pipe or in combination with other nonhabituating botanicals (see chapter 7). To make a tea for respiratory relief, add one teaspoon of seeds (they may be crushed) to a cupful of boiling water and allow to steep, covered with a loose lid to retain the vapors, for approximately ten minutes before straining. If desired, the seeds may then be chewed for their remaining essence. Honey may be added to the tea.

Cloves too are useful in relieving stomach distress, gas, nausea, vomiting, and faintness. Clove tea can be prepared by dropping five or six cloves into one-half cup of bubbling hot water. Cooled, this essence can be drunk before going to bed. Alternatively, a teaspoon of powdered cloves can be stirred into a cupful of boiling water and allowed to stand for several minutes. As is well known, cloves have long been used for their antiseptic and pain-soothing properties. Clove oil is frequently dropped into an aching tooth to relieve pain.

I have thus far described some weapons against constipation that are *ordinarily uppermost* in my mind. There are, however, many other natural remedies. Following are those I call laxative afterthoughts.

LAXATIVE AFTERTHOUGHT: Before breakfast try drinking a cupful of water as hot as can be tolerated.

LAXATIVE AFTERTHOUGHT: Combine two teaspoons of flaxseeds (bought in a health food store in the whole seed state) with a cupful of cold water. Allow the mixture to stand for half an hour prior to drinking the entire contents. Another method, evidently used for more deep-seated constipation woes, consists of swallowing one or two tablespoons of the whole seeds along with a good amount of ordinary tap water and eating some stewed prunes. Some people are even said to eat flaxseeds whole, thoroughly chewed with little or no water, to create a laxative condition.

To loosen mucus in the intestines and chest, as well as to control coughs and, hopefully, alleviate urinary or digestive problems, drop two tablespoons of flaxseeds into a quart of water. After boiling the mixture until only one-half quart remains, drink the liquid throughout the day. Interestingly, the seeds of flax are said to encourage elimination because of their swelling action in the intestinal tract. Only fully ripened seeds are sold by the health stores because immature seed pods are considered toxic.

LAXATIVE AFTERTHOUGHT: Try drinking one-half cup of basil (common or sweet) tea prepared by steeping one teaspoon of dried basil (*Ocimum basilicum*) in boiling water for about ten minutes before straining. Some have reportedly taken this dosage (one-half cup sipped slowly) two or three times during the day. In addition to relieving constipation, sweet basil is believed to have antispasmodic properties. It is also useful for fighting stomach cramps, intestinal or gastric catarrh, and nausea (including vomiting).

LAXATIVE AFTERTHOUGHT: Try drinking, throughout the day, a pint of chickweed tea. This is prepared by dropping three generous tablespoons of dried chickweed (*Stellaria media*) into one quart of water which is boiled until only one pint remains. In addition to being used as a laxative (flavored with honey), hot chickweed tea once enjoyed a reputation for relieving intestinal gas, exercising a soothing effect on mucous membranes, and expelling phlegm from the respiratory passageways. In less sophisticated times, fresh chickweed was gathered by the wayside and prepared as a substitute for spinach, using only the tender young plant sections to avoid the stringiness that comes with overmaturation.

LAXATIVE AFTERTHOUGHT: Try drinking one-half cup of red clover tea (*Trifolium pratense*) prepared by steeping two teaspoonfuls of the dried blossoms in boiling water for about ten minutes. As with basil, some people slowly sip one-half cupful of red clover tea two or three times during the day (with or without honey). The flowers (which usually appear more purplish than red) have long been alleged to be useful in stimulating sluggish livers or gall bladders, aiding the appetite, alleviating coughs, and promoting expectoration. Some believe the blossoms have antispasmodic properties valuable in fighting asthma. In the days of my bronchial misery, I often picked and thoroughly chewed the blossoms I found along the roadside. Glory to God, it flourishes wild over a wide range of North America for the taking (but to be on the safe side, wash the blossoms before chewing them).

LAXATIVE AFTERTHOUGHT: Try drinking, as directed on the label, tea made from the seeds of psyllium (*Plantago psyllium*) sold in health food stores. These seeds, as those of flax and fenugreek, contain mucilage which helps elimination. Psyllium is a member of the plantain family, common as lawn pests throughout the nation. *Plantago major*, a variety with broad leaves, is also apparently of value in the control of hay fever, is free for the taking, and when young and tender is often eaten.

I have, with no ill results, eaten plantain leaves in the raw state more or less regularly for years and believe they will one day be recognized as having a certain degree of effectiveness in the gradual control of hay fever. Tastewise, I prefer *Plantago major* to *Plantago lanceolata* (the lance-shaped narrow-leaf variety also plentiful in my yard).

Many people are allergic to plantain pollen but plantain tea seemingly has a beneficial effect on those suffering from sinusitis, coughs, colds, common hay fever and bronchitits.

LAXATIVE AFTERTHOUGHT: Agar, a seaweed known variously as agar-agar, vegetable gelatin, or Chinese gelatin, contains a gelatinous material that is soothing to an inflamed intestinal tract and antagonistic to the mucus deposits therein. Powdered agar is often sprinkled on stewed prunes, figs or other fruits for the control of constipation. According to one report, invalids are some-times given agar as an easy-to-digest, nutritive food and to relieve congested bowels.

Agar can be purchased in health food stores, where information can be obtained on how much and how often to drink it for laxative action.

Agar is also used in a number of commercial candies, ice creams and jellies. Since highly processed foods are involved in poisoning the human body by gradual de-grees, perhaps an abundant commercial use of agar powder in junk foods would unlock the bowels of Amer-ica and restore regularity on a sublime scale unknown to modern times!

Altering the body's chemical balance to the desired end can obviously not be achieved overnight. As the sys-tem gradually begins to heal itself, peculiar reactions may occur as longstanding poisons are dissolved. Some refer to such an episode as a "healing crisis."

During the six months that I gradually tapered off all respiratory medicines (August 7, 1972-February 28, 1973), I experienced several "healing crises." About six more months of drugless living then passed with pro-gressively less "crisis" and in August, 1973, I underwent my last asthma attack. (Had I known at the outset of my detoxification program what I know now, I believe I could have subdued asthma at least several months ear-lier.)

During my "healing crises" I sometimes seemed to ex-pectorate more mucus rather than less. At times, diarrhea and constipation followed one another in a peculiar cycle. Itchy rashes were not uncommon. It dawned on me at length, however, that all I needed to be as poisonous as a rattlesnake was a pair of fangs! What I was actually undergoing was the gradual elimination of toxic materials from my tortured system. I was, indeed, gradually improving even though it sometimes appeared I was growing worse.

The root cause of chronic disease is generally *body pollution*, and one does not have to attend medical school to comprehend this. In fact, medical school may be the last place one needs to go to learn the glad tidings. To be forewarned is to be forearmed, according to the old adage, and anyone who thinks Mother Nature can be abused indefinitely without striking back is not going to be around to celebrate victory over the old girl.

The detoxification program I have outlined may be modified by respiratory sufferers to suit individual tastes or situations. While other specific aids to respiratory control are absolutely vital (altered eating habits, vitamin-mineral intake, proper exercise, sufficient sleep, herbal therapy, avoidance of allergy-causing substances, withdrawal from commercial medicines), detoxification of the system is the first major objective of the campaign. As encouragement, I shall now note several detoxification benefits that gradually blessed me after several months of cautious campaigning in enemy territory.

DETOXIFICATION BENEFIT: Although the Vitamin C I was daily taking (and to some extent the

Vitamin E) may be diuretic in action taken in therapeutic volume, I was pleased to find that within four months I was having fewer kidney calls at night and was sleeping with greater ease than I had for the past five years.

DETOXIFICATION BENEFIT: After a little more than four months, my "seltzer" bottle was still half full. I was suffering less acidity and my chronic indigestion had begun to subside as my program gained momentum. In the "old days," I had consumed the effervescent, pop-pop-fizz-fizz seltzer tablets like chocolate bonbons. Had detoxification done no more for me than check acidity, it would have bordered on the divine. The garbage man got my remaining tablets.

DETOXIFICATION BENEFIT: At the outset of my campaign, in early August of 1972, my pulse frequently "raced" at rates of ninety to ninety-five beats per minute "at rest." There had, of course, been a gradual deterioration in my pulse health as the asthma (and chronic hay fever) problems increased. By December, 1972, however, my average pulse rate had dropped to approximately eighty-five to ninety beats per minute under "normal" conditions. I was able upon occasion to jog rather far (by no means recommended for everybody!) and suspected that Vitamin E (with help from Vitamin C, among others) had actually relieved the pressures on my heart at least 50 percent by improving my general circulation.

During January, 1973, I gladly noted my average pulse range was frequently seventy-two to eighty beats per minute upon coming home from the office. A few months later my pulse ranged from fifty-six to seventy-two beats per minute after leaving the office and sixty-two was not uncommon when relaxing. (Things to which I was allergic could, however, run my pulse up unduly. Cigarette smoke, dust, molds, old papers, animal dander, and offfice carbon paper were all pulse exciters, although I could tolerate tobacco smoke somewhat better by the time my last asthma attack occurred in August, 1973.) Once the body is detoxified, the sufferer should witness an improvement in pulse health irrespective of the culprit(s) involved!

DETOXIFICATION BENEFITS: During February, 1973, (six months after beginning my program), I chronicled a number of distinct detoxification benefits in addition to the diminished bronchial congestion. For example, the spots which often came before my eyes (attributed to "nerves" by doctors) had become less bothersome. Fever blisters, once almost constant it seemed, had become rare and my lips did not chap or crack painfully as before. Even the heels of my feet, which were previously quite rough, had become almost as smooth as a baby's leg. Cracks atop the big toes and on the fingers, which had particularly plagued me during cold weather, had begun to yield in a definite way as my metabolism improved.

I noted a decrease in earaches as well as in the ear "ringings" and "poppings" that vex many mucus-saturated respiratory sufferers. Raw sore throats declined in number too. (While slippery elm tablets seemed to help, I still believe that gargling with Listerine is effective, notwithstanding the advertising restrictions placed upon the manufacturer by the FDA.)

Also during the course of my detoxification victories, my "nerves" were much less "frayed." Undoubtedly, then, any enhancement in general health is bound to help the nervous system. Equally welcome, general fatigue ceased to trouble me.

DETOXIFICATION BENEFIT: I mention a very painful hemorrhoidal condition last since it yielded considerably slower than the other problems discussed. My physician had indicated that it would be necessary to relieve me of several inches of my lower intestinal tract after the bloody stools, assorted pains and ungodly itchings had, presumably, driven me mad. As I halfheartedly awaited the coming knife, my respiratory program began to slowly aid the hemorrhoids as well. After several years of strict compliance with my regimen, I felt that I was on the way to permanent relief from the accursed hemorrhoidal miseries.

As for weaponry, I used a basic multivitamin-mineral capsule which contains 10,000 International Units of Vitamin A and 5 milligrams of Vitamin B6 (pyridoxine). To these I daily added approximately 30,000 International Units of Vitamin A (for a total of 40,000 I.U., just under the toxic level), 100 to 150 milligrams of B6 (check toxicity, if any), and a few calcium tablets because I had reduced my use of milk products. I was also taking additional Vitamin E and Vitamin C daily. However I think B6, a muscle-nerve-antihistamine vitamin of great promise, may have been the key weapon in this arsenal.

Apart from this, it should be emphasized that constipation is the mortal enemy of hemorrhoids (or piles) and straining upon the commode must definitely be avoided. As mentioned before, the addition of two teaspoons of bran to the diet three times daily is considered of value in overcoming constipation. On the other hand, large amounts of bran can be antagonistic to piles, as are hard, frequent coughs and obesity.

Whatever the theories on roughage or fiber intake, I personally feel that, notwithstanding any momentary high-fiber "wear or tear" that may have occurred, my own best results did not come until I began regularly eating two completely raw meals daily and part of a third.

Good health is more to be sought than all this suffering world's treasures. Once our systems are properly detoxified, we will find a measure of relief (often incredible) for many, many ailments—including hemorrhoids.

CHAPTER V

FORMULATING A VITAMIN-MINERAL SUPPLEMENT PROGRAM

On the same red-letter day that I began taking Vitamin E, I also purchased vitamin tablets containing 5,000 International Units of Vitamin A, 400 International Units of Vitamin D, 2 milligrams of B1, 2.5 milligrams of B2, 1 milligram of B6, 1 microgram of B12, 50 milligrams of Vitamin C, 50 milligrams of niacinamide, 1 milligram of pantothenic acid and 15 milligrams of iron. This comes close, I believe, to being the weakest vitamin tablet (iron being the lone mineral therein) on the market today.

I used it exclusively until January, 1973, with the exception of my *therapeutic intakes* of Vitamin E and Vitamin C (which was not increased because of false fears until about the end of November, 1972). Any progress I made vitaminwise *prior* to the latter part of January, 1973, was thus achieved with the "nontherapeutic" formula described above, Vitamin E and, finally, Vitamin C therapeutically.

Toward the end of January, 1973, I came to realize that minerals were just as vital to health as vitamins and that individuals varied in their requirements. With this in mind, I visited a local health food store and selected a jar of 100 therapeutic-strength multivitamin-mineral capsules for $1.98 (widely sold by a well-known national firm to the uninformed for about $6.50). To this formula I subsequently added any supplemental vitamins or minerals I deemed necessary after due consideration. It is my honest opinion that the therapeutic-strength multivitamin-mineral capsule is the cornerstone upon which to build a good vitamin-mineral supplement program. Before beginning any new vitamin-mineral program, consult your doctor.

The basic formula is:

Vitamin A	(palmitate synthetic)	10,000 I.U.
Vitamin D	(irradiated ergosterol)	400 I.U.
Vitamin B1	(thiamine mononitrate)	10 mg.
Vitamin B2	(riboflavin)	10 mg.
Vitamin B6	(pyridoxine hydrochloride)	5 mg.

Vitamin B12	(cyanocobalamin USP)	5 mcg.
Vitamin C	(ascorbic acid)	200 mg.
Calcium pantothenate		20 mg.
Vitamin E	(d-alpha tocopheryl acetate)	15 I.U.
Niacinamide, (B3)		100 mg.
Iron	(from ferrous sulphate)	12 mg.
Iodine	(from potassium iodide)	0.15 mg.
Manganese	(from manganese sulphate)	1 mg.
Copper	(from copper sulphate)	2 mg.
Zinc	(from zinc sulphate)	1.5 mg.
Magnesium	(from magnesium carbonate)	65 mg.

Before formulating a list of nutrients that may be of value in conquering asthma, it is necessary to know exactly what this condition is.

ASTHMA: A generally allergic, recurring condition marked by an uncontrollable, fitlike difficulty in breathing accompanied by wheezing noises due to violent but intermittent tightening of the bronchial tube muscles that are often plugged with mucus. Symptoms are a frequent cough, considerable expectoration, tightness in the chest and the feeling that one may suffocate. Because inhaled air is imprisoned in the lungs, exhaling is commonly more difficult than inhaling. This is due to a violent reaction (muscle spasms) within the smaller (usually) bronchial tubes that have been narrowed by tissue swellings and mucus accumulations that cannot be readily dislodged. Consequently, dizziness from lack of oxygen, heart poundings, nervous prostration and general debility are not uncommonly experienced.

A low blood sugar level appears characteristic and not a few asthmatics can be found with disorders of the adrenal glands as well.

An asthma attack may be brought about by colds, physical or emotional stresses, sudden weather or temperature changes, molds, mildews, old papers or books, feather pillows or mattresses, insect bites, vigorous exercising, belly laughing, sundry foods (including additives), air pollution, cigarette smoke, insecticides or other sprays, gasoline or paint fumes, medicines, all types of dust concentrations and airborne pollens.

A condition that may resemble asthma (that commonly comes with increasing years but can also affect the comparatively young) is caused by a weakened heart and is not, in all likelihood, caused by an allergy. And to complicate it all, one can suffer from asthma, bronchitis and hay fever simultaneously in various combinations.

While vitamin-mineral needs vary as a consequence of one's diet, age, size, metabolic responses, powers of assimilation, and according to the disease at hand, the following appear especially helpful in the control or cure of asthma when used faithfully:

Vitamin A	Helps to increase resistance to infection. Important for the health of the mucous membranes of the respiratory and digestive tracts. R.D.A. is 5,000 I.U. Some researchers re-

port good results with doses of 25,000 to 40,000 I.U. but toxicity can occur with doses in excess of 50,000 I.U. (Pregnant women should not take *any* Vitamin A unless prescribed by a doctor, since it is suspected of causing birth defects.) Fish-liver oil capsules appear best source outside raw vegetables (such as carrots, sweet potatoes, spinach, broccoli, kale, Brussels sprouts), liver, eggs, margarine and fortified dairy products.

Vitamin B complex

The B complex strengthens the nervous system, thus enabling the body to handle stress better. It also helps provide energy. The many members of this group are virtually always found together in the same foods. Brewer's yeast, raw fruits and vegetables, whole wheat, peanuts and oatmeal are top sources. Most B Vitamins are water soluble and are not stored in the body. Extra amounts of B2, B6, and pantothenic acid may be wise as these vitamins help form antibodies. B6 and pantothenic acid appear to have an antihistamine action.

Vitamin B2
(Riboflavin)

Helps form antibodies. Also combats eye malfunctions and irritations. Vital in cell respiration. Found in milk, whole grain products, liver, green vegetables, eggs. No known toxicity by mouth. I found 25 milligrams daily (in addition to my basic vitamin capsule) ample.

Vitamin B6
(Pyridoxine)

Helps form antibodies. Necessary for fat, protein and carbohydrate metabolism. Appears to have definite muscle-nerve and antihistamine properties. Found in beef liver, fish, bananas, cabbage, raisins, wheat germ, peanuts, walnuts. Check toxicity, if any. I used between 50 and 150 milligrams daily in addition to the amount contained in my basic vitamin capsule.

Vitamin B12
(Cyanocobalamin)

Helps maintain a healthy nervous system. Also necessary for formation of blood cells and of value in treatment of pernicious anemia.

Found in liver, shellfish, Camembert cheese. No known oral toxicity but addition of 25 micrograms daily would appear sufficient.

Pantothenic Acid   Major role is in enzyme system, particularly production of energy. Believed useful in combating exhaustion of the adrenal glands and in fighting bronchial asthma and hay fever in some individuals. While no experimental side effects are known (except in doses of 10,000 milligrams or more), addition of only 50 to 150 milligrams daily at various times would apparently aid some persons.

Calcium pantothenate (a "salt" of pantothenic acid) is required in the synthesis of antibodies and, like pantothenic acid, aids the adrenal glands.

While much pantothenic acid is destroyed in the milling of flour, it is found in beef, kale, broccoli, avocados, split peas, lentils, lima beans, cashew nuts, egg yolks.

Vitamin C   Vitamin C aids asthmatics by neutralizing histamines, fighting bacterial infections, and combating stress. Generally, it is necessary for integrity of capillaries; growth and development of blood vessels, teeth, bones, other tissues; for wound healing. Also important for healthy functioning of adrenal gland and pituitary gland. It increases the absorption and utilization of iron (when taken together).

I take 2,000 to 3,000 milligrams throughout the day, split into doses of 500 milligrams each, which are slightly chewed and swallowed with little or no water. This seems to be the best method to control hay fever for me. (The mouth can be later rinsed with water to avoid acid stain, if any, to teeth.) I have had no colds since commencing this regimen and would not hesitate to increase my intake by several thousand milligrams per day if threatened by a cold or confronted by an unexpected hay fever difficulty. After the medicines were finally purged from my system, I noticed the antihistamine powers of Vitamin C were definitely stronger.

Because Vitamin C cannot be stored in the body, it is necessary to replenish it on a daily basis for optimum results. Moreover, heat destroys Vitamin C quite rapidly and raw foods are thus all the more vital (especially citrus fruits, spinach, tomatoes). As with Vitamins A, B complex and possibly E, the value of Vitamin C in fighting respiratory ailments or "allergies" will ultimately be made manifest if faithfully tested.

Vitamin D

Necessary for development of bones and teeth.

Maximum single dose purchasable without prescription is 400 I.U. I take 800 - 1200 I.U. daily (5,000 I.U. claimed possibly toxic in some persons taken over prolonged periods of time). Sun is preferred source and cod-liver oil or other fish-liver oils are considered excellent too but cod-liver oil may not be tolerated by persons with gall bladder or other digestive ailments.

Vitamin E

Functions as an antioxidant. Reportedly protects against the effect of pollution on the respiratory system.

Vitamin E is described as essentially nontoxic by some researchers, although doses of 4,000 I.U. or more have produced side effects in some persons. Individuals suffering from chronic *rheumatic* heart disease could be fatally stricken by ingesting Vitamin E without *strict* medical supervision, and those with high blood pressure or diabetes should take Vitamin E only with the consent of their doctors. (Please see comments in chapter 1 on the therapeutic use of vitamin E.)

I often took from 400 to 800 International Units daily until my asthma was vanquished and thereafter reduced my intake to 400 I.U. daily. I found Vitamin E more effective when combined with Vitamins A, B complex, C, and F, as well as the mineral manganese (which some researchers believe may aid in the treatment of asthma. Check with your doctor first though as this mineral affects blood sugar). Like Vitamins A and

C, Vitamin E is of particular value to respiratory sufferers because it promotes the body's resistance to viral infections. If it did no more than protect the lungs against air pollution it would be a godsend.

Vitamin E is found especially in wheat germ, whole grains, wheat germ oil, vegetable oils, green vegetable leaves, soybeans, raw seeds or nuts, milk, eggs, meats and margarine. (Vitamin E and iron are incompatible, so if iron is taken in the form of vitamin-mineral tablets, it should be taken 6-8 hours before or after the Vitamin E.)

Vitamin F
(Unsaturated
Fatty Acids)

This vitamin helps destroy cholesterol deposits, is vital in promoting normal gland function (particularly the thyroid and adrenal glands) and aids in the circulation of oxygen to vital organs, cells and tissues. Excellent sources are raw seeds; wheat germ; and vegetable oils such as peanut, soybean, and corn.

Vitamin P
(Bioflavonoids)

Aids in the proper absorption of Vitamin C, protects against infections, prevents hemorrhaging of cells, blood vessels and connective tissues. Best sources are the white inner pulp of citrus fruits and peelings but also found in apricots, cherries, grapes, plums, rose hips, blackberries, and buckwheat. No known toxicity.

Bone Meal
(Calcium)

Asthmatics who have reduced their intake of milk products may need several bone meal tablets daily in order to maintain strength of bones and aid heart, muscle, nerve and blood clotting functions. Calcium also aids in the body's use of iron, a lack of which reduces the blood's oxygen-carrying ability, often resulting in difficulty in breathing as well as fatigue.

From 800 to 1,400 milligrams needed daily according to age and size. While one cup steamed collard greens has 376 milligrams of calcium, steamed dandelion greens 252, steamed turnip greens 267 and steamed mustard greens 193, respectively, most vegetables rank quite low in calcium and fruits even less.

Calcium absorption is very dependent upon the presence of Vitamins A, C and D, as well as iron, phosphorus, protein intake and certain body acids. However, foods containing oxalic acid in undue volume (especially rhubarb, beet greens, lamb's quarters, spinach, Swiss chard, purslane or chocolate) can retard calcium absorption. Eating excessive amounts of such foods may possibly cause kidney or gall bladder stones in some persons when the calcium combines with too much oxalic acid.

Moreover, in some persons an oversupply of Vitamin D and calcium (though normally indispensable to one another!) may bring about undue tissue or bone calcification. Body acids of normal type are needed to prevent the calcium from concentrating in tissues or joints. Older people, or individuals with insufficient hydrochloric acid secretions, may prefer to obtain additional calcium from dolomite tablets instead of bone meal. Oddly, at times, calcium may lessen the need for Vitamin C.

Kelp

Seaweed is of benefit in maintaining the mucous membranes and is thus of value in fighting respiratory ills.

I take six 10-grain kelp tablets before retiring without fear despite the Food and Drug Administration's recommendation of only one tablet daily containing 0.15 milligram of iodine. One 10-grain kelp tablet also contains 2 milligrams of organic iron (10 milligrams recommended for men and 18 for women. Iron may be toxic in some individuals if 100 milligrams are ingested daily over a prolonged period). However, iron is ordinarily absorbed by the body in about four hours and not only aids in the transportation of oxygen in the blood stream but helps control colitis, constipation, anemia, labored breathing, paleness of skin, brittle nails, internal hemorrhaging associated with peptic ulcers, and fatigue.

Iron may, in some instances, interfere with Vitamin E's absorption. Some scientists claim the opposite however, particularly when the body contains sufficient Vitamin C, calcium, hydrochloric acid. Just to be on the safe side, let 6-8 hours elapse between the ingestion of Vitamin E and the ingestion of iron (in the form of a vitamin-mineral capsule or tablet).

In addition to organic or natural salts and iodine, kelp seaweed tablets (depending on the source) are alleged to contain not only some 21 amino acids so vital to the digestive processes but over 12 vitamins and possibly 60 minerals including copper, potassium, cobalt, magnesium, manganese, calcium, chlorine, sulphur and zinc.

It is available in powdered form for use as a salt substitute on foods. Some health centers even sell dulse and Irish moss seaweed herbal teas.

Manganese

Some researchers believe manganese may possibly be of some value in fighting asthma because of its role in balancing blood sugar. (Asthmatics generally have low blood sugar.) I found that 5 milligrams, twice daily, a few weeks at a time, was of some aid to me in my battle with asthma, especially when I took it in combination with Vitamins E, B complex and C. No RDA (Recommended Daily Allowance) has been established yet, but the average daily need is probably from 3 to 9 milligrams. Doses as high as 60 milligrams are sold without a prescription but manganese is easily absorbed and *large intakes are not normally prescribed or recommended.* Manganese works with B1, calcium, phosphorus and, importantly, Vitamin E. Its largest concentrations are found in the liver, bones, pituitary gland and the pancreas. However, a lack of manganese may contribute to hearing loss, ear noises, paralysis, convulsions, blindness and dizziness in certain individuals. Raw green vegetables, whole-grain products, egg yolks, legumes, pineapples and raw seeds or nuts are considered excellent natural sources.

Potassium

Appears to have a role in aiding respiratory performance of asthmatics by stabilizing activity of the adrenal glands so they can produce natural antihistamine-type cortisone and adrenal secretions. (This way, the asthmatic can avoid the toxic, synthetic, adrenalinelike drugs used by allergy doctors such as ephedrine, adrenaline, cortisone and Isoproterenol.) When the adrenal glands are placed under stress because of the asthmatic's typically low-blood sugar level, an increased volume of potassium is lost in the urine. If potassium is truly an antihistamine element, as some researchers claim, more study should be accorded it in this respect. However, potassium is also vital in such things as heart muscle activity, nervous system health, and kidney performance.

Potassium gluconate believed to be the easiest form to absorb, but potassium tablets should *not* be taken in excess of container labels. No complete agreement on body's daily requirements, but it's thought that the average person's daily intake is 2,000-2,500 milligrams. I, personally, think *all* the asthmatic's (or other allergy sufferer's) potassium needs should be derived naturally from low-salt *raw* vegetables, dried or raw fruits, raw sunflower seeds, peanuts, bean sprouts, whole-grain products.

Miscellaneous Supplements

Garlic, which has been used throughout history as an aid against asthma, bronchitis, influenza, tuberculosis, catarrh, whooping cough, wheezing, choking coughs, nasal infections, laryngitis, sinusitis, diptheria, and common colds, contains an active natural antibiotic called allicin that annihilates germs without any of the side effects of modern bactericides or antiseptics. Several garlic cloves can be eaten daily. (The fumes are allegedly moderated by chewing fresh parsley leaves or roots with them.) Better yet, consider consuming two or three parsley-garlic capsules at each meal as this scientifically prepared supplement is said to leave no aftereffects odorwise and is convenient to take.

Pollen tablet supplements may also hold some promise as an antihistamine agency in combating asthma (or hay fever) if taken with regularity. (See chapter on honey.)

The individual asthma (or chronic bronchitis) sufferer will, of course, have to carefully determine how many, if any, of the nutrients discussed can be profitably added to the suggested basic multivitamin-mineral formula previously outlined. It should be noted that the suggested early-fight daily intake of 40,000 International Units of Vitamin A *includes* the 10,000 International Units already present in the suggested basic capsule.

Under normal conditions, Vitamin A builds strong teeth and bones; aids digestion; promotes healthy skin; repairs tissues or membranes throughout the body (thus protecting the eyes, nose, mouth, throat, lungs, intestinal tract, kidneys); combats bacteria, infections, and air pollution. A lack of Vitamin A is manifested in eye sites; night blindness; defective teeth; rough, prematurely aged, dry or scaly skin; loss of appetite or smell; frequent feelings of fatigue; diarrhea; and an increased likelihood of infections.

On the other hand, symptoms of Vitamin A *toxicity* are appetite loss; nausea; vomiting; diarrhea; blurred vision; skin rashes; itchy or peeling skin; hair loss; deep pain in one's bones or bone fragility; headaches; decreased thyroid activity; liver or spleen enlargement; sore lips, dry or flaky skin; irritabilty; and fissuring of the mouth at the corners. One can apparently have some of the *same* symptoms when suffering from a longstanding deficiency of Vitamin A as when one ingests too much Vitamin A. (Vitamin A is stored in the body and the Recommended Daily Allowance is usually 5,000 I.U. for adults.)

If the symptoms of toxicity are correctly diagnosed, they disappear within a few days after discontinuance of Vitamin A. Upon resumption of intake, of course, one selects a dosage in line with his own absorption level. Reportedly, in cases where no Vitamin A deficiency exists, a daily intake of 50,000 International Units *could prove toxic*, but as much as 100,000 International Units have been given by physicians for relatively *short periods of time under close observation.* It appears *most cases of toxicity occur in individuals taking 100,000 I.U.* of Vitamin A *daily for many months.* The safe therapeutic level for those deficient in Vitamin A lies somewhere between 25,000 I.U. and 50,000 I.U. daily.

In order to be on the safe side, I lowered the 50,000 I.U. maximum to 40,000 I.U. daily after my last asthma attack. From there I tapered the dose down to 20,000 I.U. daily (including the 10,000 I.U. in my basic vitamin capsule).

People do not appear to be adversely affected by the regular consumption of fried beef liver which may contain in excess of 240,000 I.U. of Vitamin A in a single pound (uncooked). A cupful of diced cooked carrots contains an estimated 15,750 I.U. of Vitamin A, whereas one large raw carrot has about 11,000 I.U. of carotene which is converted by the body into Vitamin A. Sweet potatoes vary in Vitamin A content according to the darkness of the flesh (the darker ones contain the most). However, a small baked sweet potato contains an estimated 8,100 I.U. of Vitamin A.

As noted earlier, I place great stock in the regular consumption of raw sweet potatoes and carrots in the fighting of asthma, bronchitis and hay fever. So far as I was ever able to discern, I never turned orange or yellow from this regimen. There have been several cases recorded of carrot fiends who contracted a condition called xanthosis, a yellowish discoloration of the skin brought about by hypercarotenemia. It is estimated that one ounce of carrot juice could contain as much as 5,000 I.U. of Vitamin A in the beta-carotene form. There seems little chance, however, that the average respiratory sufferer will come down with the pathological affliction called hypervitaminosis A from drinking too much carrot juice.

As mentioned earlier, the therapeutic dosage of Vitamin C is 2 to 3 grams daily (or 2,000 to 3,000 milligrams). Those who have reservations about this intake may be interested in the following defense of Vitamin C by the renowned Dr. Linus Pauling in the January, 1977, issue of *The Body Forum:*

Ascorbic acid has only a small value in providing protection against colds when it is given in low doses. Its effectiveness goes up rapidly when larger amounts are used. The regimen that I recommended in my book is 1 gram or more of Vitamin C per day with one or two grams every hour when you feel the symptoms of a cold coming on. The gram or two an hour treatment continues until symptoms disappear. Regnier in his observations found that it was best to take decreasing amounts over several days after suppressing the symptoms, to prevent them from recurring. I might add that a careful reading of the literature will disclose that Vitamin C does not cause kidney stones, destroy Vitamin B12, or cause cancer, as some have indicated. Such statements are simply inaccurate. A detailed discussion of this is found in my book. Vitamin C in large doses (3 grams or more) may have a laxative effect on some people. Generally, this effect disappears after three or four days, or if the vitamin is taken with a meal.

As is well known, Vitamin C is destroyed by air and heat. While the Recommended Daily Allowance can range as low as 35 milligrams for infants under six months, the RDA for lactating mothers is estimated to be 80 milligrams daily and for adults 45. Many studies have demonstrated that the body's Vitamin C level is lowered more rapidly by surgery, stress, fatigue, fevers, nicotine, noxious fumes, baking soda, and medicines of many kinds such as sulfa drugs, antibiotics, and aspirin. It is reported that one cigarette can quickly neutralize about 25 milligrams of Vitamin C. However, we should not underestimate the value of Vitamin C in lessening fatigue, preventing colds, promoting wound healing, strengthening connective tissues, aiding red blood cell formation, decreasing cholesterol in the blood stream, fighting bacterial infections of sundry origins, overcoming certain allergy-causing substances, and alleviating shortness of breath in due time.

Adverse symptoms brought about by a lack of Vitamine C include deficiencies of the bones, teeth, gums, blood vessels, digestive and respiratory systems. If side effects should occur from overuse of Vitamin C, they would probably be manifest in a slight sense of burning at the time of urination, some looseness of the bowels, or skin rashes that may, possibly, be the body's way of eliminating toxic materials quite apart from the supposed excessive intake of Vitamin C. Nonetheless, if such symptoms occur, the amount of Vitamin C taken can be adjusted.

Whatever the decision as to Vitamin C ingestion, raw citrus fruits, Brussels sprouts, collards, cauliflower, strawberries, cabbage, guavas, blackberries, currants, raspberries, tomatoes, cantaloupes, watermelons, dewmelons (honeydews), pineapples, papayas, dandelion greens, kohlrabi, leeks, sweet peppers, squash, rutabagas, kale, and potatoes can be relied upon to supply Vitamin C. Of course, the antihistamine action is hastened when Vitamin C is taken therapeutically in tablet form.

While the amount of vitamin-mineral supplements taken will vary in accordance with such factors as individual needs and general eating habits, it seems best to take the greatest amount during the largest meal. Of course, Vitamin C can be taken effectively alone throughout the day. I have, however, successfully taken Vitamin C between meals with a cup of antihistamine herbal tea such as mullein, well flavored with raw honey and supported by 25 milligrams of B2, 50 milligrams of B6, 50 milligrams of pantothenic acid, and one or two bone meal tablets to heighten the reaction. If the stomach is empty, one might want to eat several ounces of sunflower seeds which, in early times, were considered of some value in the gradual correction of respiratory ills, particularly coughs and colds. However, it seems best, as indicated, to take most supplements with the heaviest meal. Additional supplements can be taken during the other meals.

Before noting a number of nutrients that appear of some value in vanquishing bronchitis in its acute or chronic forms, here is a brief description of the general nature of this complaint.

BRONCHITIS: An inflammation of one or more of the bronchial tubes caused by infections, exposure to cold, fatigue, cigarette smoking, air pollutants, irritating substances of numerous types, or malnutrition. It is characterized by shortness of breath, muscle or back pains, chills, sore throat, coughing (at first dry but subsequently looser), feverishness, wheeziness and the frequent expectoration of phlegm as time passes on.

The *acute* form is usually more or less severe but of shorter duration, attended by fever, difficult breathing, spitting, coughing and chest pains, particularly upon coughing.

The *chronic* form is of more longstanding duration but more or less marked by a tendency to recur after periods of relative quietness. In chronic bronchitis, of course, the symptoms are more magnified. It may be complicated by other ailments and is characterized by secondary changes in tissues of the lung, sometimes quite violent coughing attacks and expectoration in both scanty and profuse stages.

A condition called bronchial asthma is caused by the spasmodic tightening of the bronchial muscles; however, chronic bronchitis is occasioned by mucus clogging the inflamed bronchial passages and when breathing becomes increasingly labored the sufferer may also experience unpleasant breath, pains in the chest, nervous exhaustion, impaired appetite, headaches, constipation and stomach disorders.

The bronchitis sufferer is said to have inflammation (or swelling) of the membranous linings of the larger bronchial tubes whereas the asthma sufferer is said to have inflammation, swelling or spasms in the smaller bronchial tubes through which air passes directly to the lungs. However, air passing through the narrowed or mucus-filled passages of the smaller bronchial tubes will generally produce a more "musical" noise (or wheeze) in the asthma victim than that encountered in the bronchitis sufferer whose drier "wheeze" appears to be more of a hissing or sizzling nature.

Bronchitis, as with asthma, may begin with seasonal complications and gradually become a year-round hardship. The exact demarcation line between asthma and bronchitis may be impossible to define, but we know that either can be the forerunner of emphysema if ineptly attended.

In the so-called "dry-cough" type of bronchitis it is exceedingly difficult to expel mucus and there seems to be no relief from the coughing spells at hand. The so-called "wet-cough" form, of course, is accompanied by an abundant discharge of mucus which is not infrequently of unpleasant color or odor.

Licorice roots, in moderation, and anise seeds, freely, have been utilized since early times for the "dry coughs," whereas wild cherry inner bark, in moderation, has been acclaimed for the "wet coughs." Since those who have chronic bronchitis are all too often nicotine addicts, they prefer to dismiss their coughing spells as "smoker's hack." Even though the poison nicotine irritates the bronchial tubes, the average smoker with bronchitis would rather flirt with the incredibly high cancer statistics and cough his head nearly off his shoulders than publicly admit the lunacy of his ways. But even after surrendering the noxious weed, the road to recovery may be fraught with hardship as a consequence of a weary system long abused.

As for nutrients needed to control or cure bronchitis in its acute or chronic forms, those previously described for asthma would seem in order for the most part. As with asthma, regular intakes for bronchitis can be adjusted in accordance with individual requirements. Of course, in due time, one can possibly reduce the daily intakes to a regular maintenance level that would probably consist of the basic multivitamin-mineral capsule described earlier, possibly bolstered with individual nutrients such as Vitamins A and D in moderate amounts on occasion, Vitamin E in accordance with personal circumstances as noted previously, bone meal tablets depending on one's current calcium intake, kelp tablets as a body conditioner, or whatever else seems indicated.

Vitamin C, I believe, should always be added daily to the basic multivitamin-mineral capsule containing 16 different nutrients, including 200 milligrams of Vitamin C, regardless of whatever additional supplements one determines to use or not use maintenancewise.

The multivitamin-mineral program at hand is intended to *gradually* revitalize the system while one's respiratory medicines are slowly discontinued. However, on occasion, the sufferer may possibly gain surprisingly quick momentary relief during respiratory attacks by testing nontoxic and nonhabituating herbal smoking formulas described further in chapter 7. For the bronchitis, asthma or hay fever sufferer with the nicotine habit, I believe it may well be possible to withdraw therefrom by regularly loading the bowl of a pipe with varying combinations of tobacco and such herbs as mullein leaves, yerba santa, coltsfoot, eucalyptus leaves, thyme, marjoram, or chamomile flowers until such time as nothing but the nonhabituating herbs are being smoked.

Having noted and described various nutrients under the specific headings of asthma and bronchitis, I shall now focus on nutrients of value in the control of hay fever (allergic rhinitis), but first I shall make a few observations regarding the variable character of this disorder.

HAY FEVER: An allergic condition, usually seasonal, characterized by prolonged sneezing, sniffing, snorting, nasal stuffiness, nervous irritabilty, occasional sinus headaches, and inflamed eyes that may, in varying degrees, itch, ache, burn, grow reddish or become tear-laden with a swollen appearance. Itching may also occur in the nose, roof of the mouth, throat and ears. The ability to hear, smell or taste may be diminished, and a hacking cough may occur if the throat becomes swollen or inflamed.

Clogged nasal passages may burn and the need to constantly wipe the nose can increase the nasal soreness that already exists. A watery, free-flowing, sticky substance (mucus) is likewise secreted in abnormal volume by the inflamed mucous membranes that line the inner surfaces of the nose and respiratory tract. If the mucus that runs so excessively from the nose drops into the lower respiratory passages in sufficient quantity, a shortness of breath resembling asthma can occur and one's sleep may be lessened.

Hay fever usually subsides or ceases altogether when the weather grows cold enough to neutralize the guilty pollens. Evidently, the rarer year-round (perennial) hay fever is caused by allergenic foods or additives, temperature changes, cosmetics, animal dander, feathers, fungus spores or molds, fabrics, furniture stuffings, air pollution, and medicines, but particularly "house dust" (which differes from outside dust). House dust is constantly loaded with allergens or toxic materials (including an allergy-causing mite or parasite of minute size) and these things are, of course, largely unaffected by outside weather conditions.

Longstanding inflammations of the sinus cavities (sinusitis) can, unfortunately, result in nasal polyps or growths in some people and it is widely estimated that approximately 30 percent of hay fever sufferers will eventually develop asthma.

However, the hay fever victim's salvation appears to lie largely in proper foods, detoxification of the system, certain herbal therapy, wholesome exercise, sunshine, fresh air to the extent possible, and in activating the body's own antibodies or antihistamine secretions to neutralize offending substances (internal or external).

As for nutrients that are useful in the control of hay fever, the sufferer may consider taking daily the basic multivatamin-mineral capsule described earlier. To this may be added the following supplements as necessary. (Please reread all previous descriptions of these nutrients.)

Vitamin A	It is probable that hay fever sufferers have had an undersupply of this membrane-healing vitamin most of their lives. I found a dosage of 30,000 I.U.'s helpful. (Beware of toxicity—please. See earlier discussion on amounts and limits.)
Vitamin B complex	Vitamins B2, B6 and pantothenic acid seem of special benefit in fighting hay fever. Taken regularly, B2 is of some aid in controlling itchy eyes, while B6 and pantothenic acid may have some value as antihistamines. Six members of the B complex family are already found in the basic capsule recommended for the main mealtime, but additional amounts (discussed earlier) may be necessary until the body is revitalized by proper eating habits.
Vitamin C	I usually take 2,000 to 3,000 milligrams throughout the day (including between meals when necessary) and even more in emergencies such as heavy ragweed fallout or threatened colds. I shall never forget the glorious sensation I had on Febru-

ary 28, 1973, when I finally reached the level where I was taking Vitamin C, in particular, as a full-time substitute for the nonassimilable drug store medicines that had systematically been wrecking my health for years.

Vitamin D

Since 400 International Units are already found in the basic capsule suggested earlier, the sufferer may want to add only 400 to 800 International Units daily and thus avoid any toxic effects. It may be that phlegm deposits are easier to cough up when Vitamin D combines with bone meal (a prime calcium and trace element source) in the body. Whatever the reason, Vitamin D works closely with Vitamin A and calcium in strengthening lung muscles and healing the mucous membranes of the respiratory system. Vitamin D also appears to work especially well with Vitamins A and C in the prevention of colds, and with calcium in the proper formation of bones and teeth. A lack of Vitamin D manifests itself in retarded growth, loss of muscular strength, abnormal heart action, unstable nervous system, and soft bones.

Vitamin E

Vitamin E may be of value in fighting hay fever because of its ability to fight air pollution and help the blood retain and circulate oxygen.

Vitamin P (Bioflavanoids)

Vitamin P appears to be interwoven with Vitamin C in the promotion of capillary vessel integrity and in fighting infections. The peels and inner white pulp of citrus fruits appear particularly loaded with Vitamin P. Consider eating, twice daily, a teaspoonful of fresh grated undyed lemon, orange or tangerine peelings flavored with several teaspoons of raw honey and fortified with B2, B6, pantothenic acid and Vitamin C. I occasionally added a little crushed bone meal and refrigerated horseradish. (The horseradish helps open the sinus passages but too much of it may pose digestive upsets for some.)

Bone Meal
(Calcium)

Two or three tablets (200 milligrams each) daily, especially for those getting insufficient calcium due to consuming less mucus-forming sweet milk may be helpful.

In evaluating these suggestions for respiratory improvement without drugs (in due time), one must guard against the mistake of believing that *any* kind of vitamin-mineral formula can replace wholesome eating habits. Manmade supplements are utilized for transforming foods into energy and for body maintenance. So far as I am aware, no claims have been advanced that they are synonymous with food. But when *properly* used, supplements are a godsend to countless people in unsound health whose eating habits are far from praiseworthy. Again, however, they are *not* synonymous with food despite all their sometimes remarkable virtues.

CHAPTER VI
HELPFUL (I TRUST) IDEAS

In my efforts to develop a program to control my asthma and hay fever, I tested a number of methods and disciplines, some of which may fill the reader with astonishment or wonder. I prefer to call them the "off-beat remedies." However, since our modern-day medical specialists seem to have a rather poor track record in curing asthma or bronchitis, and their sinus or hay fever patients often grow worse from year to year, it may well be the better part of wisdom to withold laughter as we reflect upon a little "unorthodox" therapy. Undoubtedly, in this earth-orbiting age of "medical miracles," much of the old (such as is found in homeopathy) has been unjustly scorned or foolishly abandoned in our reckless haste to be "modern." While many ailments will, of course, respond most favorably to the latest medical advances, it *may* be that *some* problems are not as complicated as the American Medical Association would lead us to suppose. Therefore, let us not condemn something merely because it is "old-fashioned" or "unsophisticated" by today's standards.

HOMEOPATHY: This is a medical system introduced by Samuel Hahnemann (1755-1843) which seeks to treat diseases by the administration of medicines in minute quantities that would produce in healthy persons symptoms similar to those of the disease. Homeopathic physicians are highly trained specialists and membership in their organizations is open to licensed physicians only.

They have at their disposal over 2,000 specially prepared medicines, predominately herbal, and they also use many natural products of mineral, animal, insect, reptilian or bacterial origin. These substances are greatly diluted and the patient is not nearly so likely to experience side effects as when treated by the average M.D.

Homeopathic physicians place considerable stock in the body's ability for self-repair. While trained in all types of medical therapy (as are other M.D.'s), homeopathic physicians will, if possible, provide a patient the opportunity to first test the amazingly harmless homeopathic medicines, dietary adjustments, proper exercise or rest programs, body massages or manipulations, and hot and cold water packs before ingesting potentially dangerous drugs currently in vogue or undergoing surgery. Fortunately, homeopathic medicines are also more economical than the "standard" ones ordinarily used, and an earnest attempt is made to diagnose illnesses in the early stages in order to prevent future inroads into the patient's health as well as his pocketbook.

If you are interested in finding a generally safer solution to many bodily ills, including respiratory problems, I recommend a remarkable book by James H. Stephenson, M.D., entitled *A Doctor's Guide To Helping Yourself With Homeopathic Remedies* (Parker Publishing Co., Inc. West Nyack, New York. Home treatment kits especially prepared for Dr. Stephenson's book are available through Similia, Inc., P. O. Box 175, Glenville Station, Connecticut 06830).

In the book, Dr. Stephenson outlines how to make various remedies. Among them is the method of preparing *Allium cepa* (the common onion), which, in high dilution, Dr. Stephenson calls his "single most effective medication for spring and fall hay fever." Following the definition for homeopathy, the onion produces in a well person the same symptoms (running, burning eyes and nose, with a profuse, watery and acrid nasal discharge) that are found in the hay fever victim! Dr. Stephenson tells us of Joseph W. who suffered each year from acute sneezing, running eyes and a dull headache but was freed of his springtime hay fever after Dr. Stephenson showed him how to prepare his own "onion medicine" in highly diluted form.

Dr. Stephenson tells of a hay fever victim who could withstand full-blown September ragweed at home but was unable to cope with the sea air while vacationing with her husband at the beach. Although she experienced untold agony *surrounded by salt water,* Dr. Stephenson cleverly administered common salt in homeopathic dilution to restore her health. As he writes in his book, "This illustrates how differently a substance acts in gross dosage, compared to its action after special preparation via homeopathic serial dilution and succession."

Anyone fortunate enough to obtain Dr. Stephenson's marvelous book will note several asthma and hay fever medicines that one should purchase from a homeopathic pharmacy instead of preparing at home. Dr. Stephenson warns us of overconfidence and reminds us that *any* condition that does not rapidly show some improvement, especially if life-threatening in nature, should be referred to a physician.

EXERCISE: Good respiratory health depends upon regular exercise. The lungs, as well as the rest of the body, cannot function properly without a certain degree of physical exertion. However, one should check with a physician if mild exercise brings about labored breathing, profuse sweating, twitching or aching limbs, chest pains or an aching heart, faintness or dizzy spells, cramps or gastrointestinal upsets. One should certainly consult a physician if unable to walk a distance of two miles.

Anyone who smokes heavily, possesses a high cholesterol level, suffers from tension or high blood pressure, has a record of heart disease in the immediate family, whose body weight is over 30 percent fat, or who is in a generally poor condition from a complete lack of exercise should visit a doctor before engaging seriously in an exercise program. (Most doctors usually see a patient in a state of rest and it would seem best to find a doctor with a treadmill facility in order to determine one's tolerance under stress conditions.)

The highball circuit devotee or table hog is likely to be in poorer physical condition than suspected and over-exertion could prove detrimental. If obesity is a problem, it is fortunate that eating a large percentage of raw foods can work wonders in due course for the average person so afflicted. And one can usually engage in moderate walking each day prior to the actual weight loss that will be necessary before engaging in a more vigorous exercise program. Fortunately, walking burns up fat and there is a tendency for the blood cholesterol and blood pressure levels to decrease. Walking not only strengthens the heart but increases the blood stream's oxygen supply and thus brings eventual relief to the respiratory sufferer.

Every person should march to his own drumbeat and find his own level of activity. Anyone in poor physical condition, needless to say, should refrain from competitive sports because the strain could conceivably prove fatal. According to many students of physical fitness, one should not engage in exercise for at least an hour after eating since exertion may hinder the digestive processes. Also, since excessively cold outside air is quite likely to be dry and could possibly absorb too much moisture from one's lungs, it may be necessary on occasion to exercise inside the home in a warm, humidified room. Boiling water on a stove or placing a pan of water atop a radiator will, to some degree, humidify or moisturize the air and loosen mucus as one exercises. Prior to exercising, one can sometimes loosen a fair amount of mucus by inhaling steam during a hot shower or even by standing near a boiling pot of water with a towel draped tent fashion over the head to catch the steam cautiously.

BREATHING EXERCISE NO. 1: Try standing militarily erect, inhaling as much air as possible without straining, and simultaneously sucking the stomach inward. Then let the breath out without straining as you bend forward (knees unbent) and touch the floor (if possible!) with your hands. Repeat several times daily and gradually increase as your endurance permits.

BREATHING EXERCISE NO. 2: Stand erect and let your arms hang beside you like a proper soldier. As you exhale as much air as possible without straining, raise your heels slowly from the floor. Then begin to inhale slowly without straining as you lift your arms from your sides until they reach directly above your head. Then exhale without straining as you slowly lower your heels and arms to the original military posture.

This lung-expanding exercise can be repeated in accordance with your endurance and, if necessary, you can breathe normally for a few seconds between the exercises.

Anyone who becomes dizzy from hyperventilation can modify this exercise and sit erect in a chair with the hands on the knees, exhaling and inhaling to the fullest extent possible short of straining.

One can devise any number of deep-breathing exercises but I personally found the above examples helpful in vanquishing my asthmatic problems, particularly when I was unable, because of adverse weather conditions, to run, jog or walk. Regular walking for considerable distances at a brisk pace is my favorite exercise although I occasionally go hiking at a leisurely pace in order to study wayside herbs or eat woodland fruits in season. I've found that deep breathing exercises can be systematically performed while walking briskly by breathing in as much air as possible and holding the breath as long as comfortably possible and then breathing out as long as possible, avoiding strain. Of course the asthmatic will not find this comfortable at first but the lungs will be strengthened as the general health improves. Breathing exercises should be stopped if one experiences dizziness and only resumed when circumstances permit.

ABDOMINAL THERAPY: The strengthening of one's abdominal muscles is particularly important since proper evacuation depends upon this. One exercise designed to improve this area consists of clasping the hands behind the neck and raising the body from a reclining position to an upright position. It may be necessary, at first, to find a way to make the legs and feet "stay down" but, in due time, the abdominal muscles should be strengthened.

WATER THERAPY: Hot water expands or opens the blood vessels while cold water contracts or shrinks them. By opening the pores, a steam bath can be helpful in eliminating uric acid or other toxic materials from an overburdened system. This in turn helps reduce the strain on one's kidneys and bladder. The hardy Finns are said to follow a steaming sauna bath by jumping into a cold lake or, during winter, rolling about in the snow. This ordeal may then be celebrated by another round of heat in the sauna bath and mercifully concluded with a dousing of cold water. While this may be a little drastic for most respiratory sufferers, some have gained relief from bronchial congestion by alternately applying hot and cold towels to the chest and back.

Some sinus or hay fever sufferers have had good results from placing cold or hot water bottles (or packs) over the sinus areas, while others have used alternate cold and hot towel applications or bathed the face in the warmest sink water endurable and then dashed cold water rapidly upon the face. If the application of heat increases the sinus pain, relief can be obtained by covering the swollen sinuses with a cold pack (in order to decrease the flow of blood therein) while simultaneously soaking the feet in a container of hot faucet water (which is said to draw blood toward the feet). If necessary, one can manufacture his own cold pack by dropping crushed ice into a plastic bag and wrapping it in a damp cloth. Experience will show you the combinations and temperatures necessary to achieve the best personal results from water therapy.

SLEEP THERAPY: Too little sleep can eventually cause or encourage many kinds of health problems but *too much* sleep can make the system sluggish and prove just as detrimental. While the sleep requirements of individuals vary, it appears that the average healthy adult needs eight hours a night. The respiratory sufferer should certainly aim for sufficient sleep in order to help rebuild his mucous membranes and general health.

The various programs discussed thus far should help make sleep more restful in due time. For example, anyone testing the vitamin-mineral program mentioned earlier should, if suffering from insomnia, benefit to some degree sleepwise. To this basic vitamin-mineral capsule can be added about 200 milligrams of magnesium as well as about 50 milligrams of pantothenic acid and several bone meal (calcium) tablets before retiring at night. These latter supplements can be taken with a glass of honey-fortified hot buttermilk or acidophilus milk (as opposed to the more mucus-forming, commercial sweet milk) about an hour before bedtime.

Breathing exercises, walks, warm showers or tub baths, music, reading, meditation, soaking the feet in hot water, or drinking hot lemonade with honey may also be helpful in relaxing the system without sleeping pills or barbiturates. Another sleeping aid is a teaspoonful of a respiratory herb such as anise seed, catnip, marjoram, skullcap or sweet balm dropped into a cup of boiling water, steeped for thirty minutes, strained, reheated, and sipped approximately one hour before retiring, fortified with raw honey for the best results. If the feet feel chilly, resting them against a hot water bottle or wearing warm socks to bed may help induce sleep. It is also good strategy to empty the bladder before trying to fall asleep.

Body pains, noise, uncomfortable bed clothing, a sagging mattress instead of a firm one, gluttony, cocoa, coffee, cola drinks, tea, salty foods that stimulate the adrenals or raise the blood pressure, direct drafts of cold or hot air upon the head while trying to fall asleep, mental anguish or tension, excitement, poor circulation, constipation, or a poorly planned sleeping schedule are just some of the things that can rob one of a sound night's sleep, not to mention house dust, airborne pollens, molds and only God knows what else. As a health tonic, however, sleep stands second to none!

ACIDOPHILUS THERAPY: Some allergy students regard sweet milk as the most mucus-forming food known. However, the Food Science Department of North Carolina State University has developed a similarly flavored but fermented product called "sweet acidophilus" that contains the valuable lactic-acid-forming bacteria known as *lactobacillus* which reportedly destroy certain harmful putrefactive intestinal bacteria that cause allergies, ulcers, and gout. Acidophilus milk is said to be as easily digested as naturally fermented yogurt and buttermilk, both of which are *lactobacillus*-laden foods that can apparently be consumed in moderation by the average respiratory sufferer without stimulating undue mucus production. Homemade yogurt or buttermilk cultures with their beneficial bacteria are natural antibiotics considered beneficial in the mastery of arthritis, constipation, diarrhea, kidney problems, and skin disorders, but the commercial preservatives found in the grocery store brands of fermented milk products may lessen their therapeutic capabilities to some degree. It is known that many of the world's oldest inhabitants include fermented milk products in their diets and seem astoundingly fit for their advanced ages.

KITCHEN THERAPEUTICS: The ordinary kitchen contains many products that are valuable as medications or treatments as well as being essential as foods.

The highly astringent unripe berries and roots of the BLACKBERRY bush have been boiled in water (with or without honey) since Biblical times and gargled to relieve a sore throat. The CHIVE, less pungent than its cousins garlic or onion, not only has an antiseptic effect on the system but has long been acclaimed (especially if consumed with honey) as helpful in subduing asthma, bronchitis, colds and coughs. CINNAMON, of some value as an antiseptic, can be brewed into an astringent tea and fortified with lemon juice and honey for ordinary colds and various bronchial complaints.

The CLOVE, mainly utilized to aid the action of other herbs and widely noted for its potent antiseptic or germicidal powers, seemingly stimulates beneficial expectoration in bronchial ailments. Several cloves can be chewed with good effect if undue tickling occurs in the throat. (The swallowing of juice derived from chewing a bit of ginseng root or slippery elm inner bark can also allegedly relieve tickling throats but, of course, one does NOT swallow the root or bark materials after the juice has been extracted.)

COFFEE, especially if taken strong on an empty stomach, may possibly be of some aid to breathing during an asthma attack because its active ingredient, caffeine, has been known to dialate bronchial tubes on occasion. CRANBERRY juice mixed with honey in equal parts and taken at the rate of one tablespoonful four to six times daily may well prove a praiseworthy mucus fighter. Pure cranberry juice was long acclaimed by early New Englanders as helpful in reducing asthma spasms, fevers, and high blood pressure. The CURRANT, a small acid fruit of the gooseberry family, may be simmered (but not boiled) for some ten minutes at the rate of two rounded teaspoons of fresh berries (or one teaspoon if dried) in a pint of water and used as an antiseptic gargle for a hoarse or sore throat. Throat lozenges, containing currant properties, were found in drug stores in bygone days.

The DATE, a veritable storehouse of nutrients, can be substituted as a candy by those respiratory sufferers addicted to sugar products. As with the fig, the date has valuable laxative properties useful in the detoxification of the system. The FIG, though high in calories like the date, is another nutrient-packed fruit that should be employed by those in the thrall of unnatural sweets. Several ounces of figs can be boiled for about ten minutes in a pint of water and the liquid sipped as desired to soothe

the respiratory passages during a cold. There are also re-ports of figs being boiled in barley water and the tea sip-ped for pulmonary disorders. For asthma and coughing spells, early Americans in the lower South reportedly boiled a pound of figs in a quart of water for five min-utes, placed them in cheesecloth, squeezed out all the juice possible, added the juice of two or three lemons, fortified the mixture with raw honey, and drank the brew as needed.

Raw GARLIC, or its cousin the ONION, thoroughly chewed, sometimes brings a measure of antiseptic relief from the woes of asthma or bronchitis. Early physicians are said to have made effective respiratory medicines by pressing juice from garlic cloves or onions and adding honey thereto. Indeed, one teaspoon of garlic juice was often given with a teaspoonful of warmed honey for asthma, coughs or common colds. Needless to say, honey renders garlic more palatable. Syrup of garlic can be made by dropping one-half pound of fresh garlic cloves. finely sliced, into one pint of boiling water. This is permitted to stand in a closed container for about twelve hours. Honey is added and the mixture is stirred until a syrupy consistency is attained. To moderate the sharp odor, a few caraway and fennel seeds may be crushed, briefly boiled in several ounces of *pure* (juice-derived) apple cider vinegar, and the seeds and liquid both stirred into the syrup of garlic. A spoonful of this concoction can be taken several times daily for asthma, bronchitis, hoarseness, chronic coughs, or digestive upsets. The leftover garlic residue can be thoroughly chewed for any "essence" remaining and this is said to somewhat reinforce the medicinal action of the garlic syrup.

Individuals experiencing continual sneezing fits have reportedly brought these episodes under control by the regular consumption of garlic. Of course, sneezing is ordinarily the body's attempt to rid itself of unwanted mucus accumulations, often toxic to the system, and certain sneeze-preventing inhalants undoubtedly have an abnormal drying effect on the nasal membranes and lungs. In fact, several aerosol nebulizer products were withdrawn from the market because of adverse side effects. What appeared at first to be prompt relief was followed by increasing respiratory irritations and rebound swellings that were worse than the initial complaints. At this point, a physician is likely to try even more dangerous "therapy" such as aristocort, celestone, decadron, haldrone, meticorten, or prednisone, all *cortisone* derivatives, the continued use of which can produce serious side effects.

GINGER root, grated, steeped in boiling water, and sweetened with honey, may be sipped by the cupful several times daily for asthma, bronchitis or colds. The root is often chewed "as is" and the juice swallowed to relieve a cough or sore throat. The GUAVA, in some parts of the world, has long been brewed along with several of the plant parts into a syrup for asthma or bronchitis.

HONEY can be taken as hot as bearable at the rate of one teaspoonful every fifteen minutes for asthma spasms, particularly if no other aid is available. An early remedy called for thorougly beating the white of an egg and mixing honey and lemon juice into it until a syrupy consistency was obtained. This formula was then taken by the teaspoonful as necessary for hoarseness. Or the whites of two eggs could be vigorously beaten with four ounces of honey-sweetened water for gargling when hoarse.

For persistent coughing, boil a cup of honey, the juice of one lemon, a pinch of cinnamon, and one-half cup of pure olive oil for about six minutes, stirring vigorously all the while to attain a uniform mixture. A teaspoon of this mixture every hour or two should convince you of its praiseworthiness. For bronchitis, try mixing a cupful each of honey, boiling water and olive oil (with a pinch of ginger added). Take four tablespoons of this upon arising, another four around midday and four more before retiring at night.

HORSERADISH, though said to possibly cause diarrhea or night sweats if consumed in excess, is claimed to be of gradual benefit for all sorts of respiratory problems, particularly if combined with raw honey and bolstered with lemon juice. For nasal blockage or stuffiness, some sufferers mix four ounces of *fresh* horseradish (finely grated) with the juice of one lemon. A teaspoon (or less) of this formula is *fully chewed* about twice daily, preferably an hour before or after eating. (This concoction should be stored in the refrigerator.) Refrigerated horseradish (purchased in the supermarket) may be used as well as fresh, but do not use frozen horseradish.

The LEEK, which many find easier to tolerate than garlic or onion, was praised in bygone days as worthy in the alleviation of bronchial congestion. It can be consumed raw or slightly steamed in salads. LEMON juice, dropped into honey-fortified sage tea and used as a gargle, will help heal a sore throat, according to some reports. If no other remedy is available, a tablespoonful of lemon juice every fifteen minutes may give comfort to some asthma and bronchitis sufferers. For bronchitis, some advocate swallowing a teaspoon or more of lemon juice and olive oil promptly upon arising each morning. In proportion to weight, the lemon may actually be the most valuable fruit the respiratory sufferer can have in his arsenal. The LIME, a relative of the lemon, apparently has many of the same virtues. MANGO juice is still consumed in a number of quarters for bronchial disorders.

ONION juice combined with honey has a long history as a home remedy for coughs, colds, and hoarseness. Eating *raw* onions regularly may not endear one to his friends but there does appear to be truth in the old claim that they are of value in vanquishing bronchitis, catarrh, coughs and the common cold. (However, garlic is claimed superior on the whole.) Boiled onions have also been praised since early times for relieving the common cold. A syrup, derived from boiling finely cut onions and honey together in a little *pure* apple cider vinegar, should be of value to some asthmatic sufferers as well as for bronchitis. Onions have also been mixed with garlic for the alleviation of circulatory and pulmonary complaints.

ORANGE peelings (as well as those of the lemon, lime or grapefruit) can be finely cut or grated, soaked for several days in pure apple cider vinegar and cooked in honey (after draining off the vinegar) until a candy-like stage is reached. This concoction can be refrigerated and several teaspoons eaten daily for relief of hay fever. Be sure you use UNDYED peels. For better results, add Vitamins C, D, E, A, B complex (particularly B2, B6 and pantothenic acid) as reinforcement.

PINEAPPLE juice has long been regarded as a natural remedy for sore throats but it appears the fresh juice is superior to the canned and one should thus endeavor to eat the fresh fruit in season. POMEGRANATE seeds have apparently been cooked into a syrup since ancient times to comfort irritated mucous membranes. Two tablespoons of the rind can be dropped into a pint and a half of water, boiled until a pint remains, allowed to cool, strained and gargled to relieve a sore throat.

TURNIP juice, boiled in honey, was long used in Russia to treat bronchitis, coughs, and colds. As for further ROOT THERAPY, the juices of horseradish and garlic are said to work more efficiently for some asthma or bronchitis sufferers if taken regularly in small amounts with the juices of beets and carrots. I have heard stories that early settlers claimed that shallow breathing, accompanied by hoarseness and a ringing cough could be relieved by taking a tablespoonful or less of red beet juice every few minutes. Moreover, a cough syrup was prepared in earlier days by cooking a good sized grated beet in pure apple cider vinegar and raw honey.

Of course, there are other KITCHEN THERAPEUTICS that may equal or excel these but I hope that I have piqued your curiosity, supplied a number of natural remedies, and stimulated you to think of ordinary substances in terms of their health-restoring powers.

SEASHORE THERAPEUTICS: As is well known, some respiratory sufferers notice an improvement in their condition when living or vacationing near salt water. I have heard that the Chinese not only go to the seaside to help their sinus problems but actually to gargle fresh, warm (not hot) seashore salt water as a top-flight method of cutting throat phlegm. It is maintained that sea water "spoils" quickly and cannot be transported inland with success. If boiling ruins the therapeutic properties of sea water as claimed, there would evidently be no way to "can" it for marketing. The Chinese also mix certain herbs with the fresh salt water and obtain even better results in treating their throat or sinus ailments. If I ever develop a throat problem while visiting the seacoast, I shall be tempted to test the gargling remedy and even sniff some sea water up my nasal passages. Meanwhile, I plan to try smoking catnip or mullein leaves, gargling one-half teaspoon of common table salt in eight ounces of warm water, chewing slippery elm inner bark and licorice roots without leaving the city limits.

NASAL POLYPS: On occasion sinus cavities become chronically swollen, inflamed, congested with phlegm and blocked by the formation of polyps that may close the nasal passages completely. Physicians often remove swollen or infected polyps surgically in order to drain the sinuses, or give the sufferer relief by a light cauterization (searing or burning) of the nasal area involved.

I don't know how frequently such delicate operations must be undertaken but I do thank God that I never carried through with my intention of seeking a "nasal operation." While I had a long and miserable history of blocked sinus passages, I do not know that I really had any nasal polyps. However, after practicing many of the self-help therapeutics described in this book, I told an ear-eye-nose-throat doctor at some length how I had gradually vanquished my asthma attacks and was comfortably controlling my once chronic hay fever problems. I made particular reference to the considerable relief received from smoking the nontoxic, nonhabit-forming herbal formulas I had carefully devised.

At this point, I asked the physician to examine my nasal passages for any signs, past or present, of nasal polyps. Finally, after a very close inspection, he announced, "Well, if you ever had any you've dissolved them." As indicated, I do not really know that I ever had any nasal polyps but I certainly had what appeared to be the usual *symptoms* for many years.

Not long ago I heard of a woman who allegedly had 130 polyps removed in the course of seven operations. Then, after developing a new supply, she reportedly "cured" them by "taking just about every vitamin in the book." She consumed daily 1,500 milligrams of Vitamin C, the bioflavonoids (particularly rutin) and brewer's yeast and lecithin.

Some people have reportedly cured sinus infections with an antiseptic garlic solution made by crushing two cloves of garlic in a garlic press. About forty drops of water (use an eyedropper) are mixed with the garlic juice and thoroughly stirred. Let this stand for a while. The sufferer then tilts his head back, squirts ten drops into each nostril, sniffs somewhat, and pinches his nose with his fingers to prevent the solution from escaping. For a few seconds, however, there is said to be an intense burning sensation, a watering of the eyes, and a flash of red light inside the head. Naturally, anyone with cataract symptoms, etc., should not attempt the "garlic grenade" therapy. (Note: garlic juice is marketed.)

NOSE FILTERS: Some years before I commenced the regimen of which I now write, Al Fort of Raleigh, North Carolina, received sinus relief by using a nose plug containing two small filter cloths (one for each nostril of course) upon which he quite ceremoniously squirted a pink chemical solution. This inspired me so that I rushed out and had myself scientifically fitted with a device similar to his. The words *nasal filter* were printed in large letters on the front lid of my official $15 kit, along with the angelic phrase *scientifically cleans the air you breathe.*

At that time, I had hay fever so strong (including asthma that later grew worse) that the introduction of a nasal filtering device had little positive effect. In fact, my drainage was so steady that I would no more than insert one set of filter cloth "mats" (properly oiled as instructed!) into the nose plug than it became necessary to replace them. The instructions on the nasal filter case had led me to believe a daily change of filter cloths in the nose plug would suffice and that one "tube" of the filter "mats" or cloths should last at least one hay fever season.

Aside from wearing a gas mask, the use of a properly fitted nose plug would seem to be a clever way to diminish the effects of pollen or dust in the air. Inasmuch as we are all somewhat differently constituted, perhaps a filtering device could aid some individuals, particularly those with milder cases. Indeed, one occasionally sees a chronic sinusitis or hay fever sufferer wearing one of those white surgical masks at certain seasons. But since the only way to achieve genuine overall results is to remove the causes of respiratory malfunctions from within, the nose plug is by no means the solution for the majority of sufferers. (And for whatever it is worth, I observed that the nose plug gave my uniformly constructed English-type nose a somewhat flat and broad aspect, not unlike that of a rain forest gorilla. Nonetheless, I would have borne the transformation with dignity had the device served me as it had my friend Fort.)

DUST PROOFING: Arthur F. Coca, M.D. reports that patients with all sorts of respiratory problems as well as those suffering from headaches, eczema, high blood pressure and arthritis have been helped by a product known as Dust-Seal (sold by L. S. Green, 160 West 59th Street, New York, N.Y.). This product, according to Dr. Coca, is a tidy, long-lasting, nonsticky, dust-catching marvel made from a "highly diluted milk-white emulsion" that one applies to mattresses, pillows, carpets, rugs, cushions, upholstered furniture and other household furnishings.

Dr. Coca says rugs thoroughly treated with Dust-Seal give protection from house dust for nearly five years despite heavy use and notes only one instance of an allergic reaction to Dust-Seal itself. While several cases were reported of sensitivity to dust-proof plastic covers, Dr. Coca speaks well of this therapy also and, amazingly, believes that over 50 percent of the population manifests sensitivity of some type to house dust!

Dr. Coca is convinced his patients had better results from using Dust-Seal than from the expensive special air conditioning equipment with filtering devices designed to rid the atmosphere of house dust and pollens. Of course, the air conditioning and central heating systems that are ordinarily sold can actually spread allergy-causing dusts, pollens, and molds. One device to combat this is called an electrostatic precipitator. This is said to filter over 95 percent of the dust from a room at the same time an ordinary, less expensive air conditioner is circulating all manner of dust, etc., about the home. While the electrostatic air filter may be a godsend for some respiratory sufferers, it should be cleaned monthly since the grid catches considerable dust, pollen or other matter and a dirty grid is said to be a possible fire hazard.

MORE NASAL OBSERVATIONS: Homes that are too hot in the winter can cause nasal stuffiness as the atmosphere becomes excessively dry. However, a regularly cleaned humidifier added to the heating system or placed in the bedroom may help. On the other hand, when there is too much summertime humidity, a dehumidifier has been known to relieve blocked nasal passages. As can be seen, the human nose undergoes great stress trying to regulate the air it breathes. Furthermore, fear of all kinds, worry, or undue excitement may possibly increase nasal blockage in "high strung" individuals. Sudden atmospheric changes, emotional upsets, industrial pollutants, to name a few, also increase the flow of blood in the nasal linings which in turn causes excessive swelling, sneezing and a flow of watery mucus.

At this point the sufferer may reach for a decongestant nose spray to shrink the swollen nasal passageways. This often immobilizes the very small protective cilia (hairs) inside the nostrils that *fight* invading dust or foreign matter—particularly when revitalized by correct living habits—and after the nose spray treatment has worn off, the rebound swelling may well be worse than that initially encountered. Needless to say, cigarette smoke, hair sprays, perfumes, fresh paint and countless other irritants will only aggravate the symptoms. One can only hope that sinus infection (i.e., a yellowish thick nasal discharge) does not set in and necessitate treatment with potent antibiotics.

Studies have found that the intestinal lining of one suffering from chronic constipation is pale of hue and, not uncommonly, swollen in the same manner noted in the nose lining of one suffering from chronic nasal blockage. Would one, therefore, be inaccurate in referring to chronic nasal blockage as constipation of the proboscis?

Momentary relief from nasal stuffiness is attained by some while engaged in vigorous exercise but shortly thereafter the stuffiness returns as a general rule.

Some clogged nose sufferers have obtained relief from dry or even cracked nasal membranes by rubbing a small amount of pure Vaseline petroleum jelly inside the nose.

In my studies, I found that one should never blow a congested nose with the mouth closed since this puts pressure upon the inner ear and very probably contributes to one's sinus-influenced earaches or ear noises. By blowing only one nostril at a time, cold germs could also be forced into the sinuses or inner ear. It is thus best to blow both nostrils simultaneously with the mouth open. Moreover, one should refrain from blowing the nose loudly or harshly in a manner suggestive of a foghorn or wild goose.

Nose breathing should also be cultivated by the respiratory sufferer who has become a habitual "mouth breather." Of course, man was designed to breathe through the nose instead of the mouth and, by learning to breathe deeply from the diaphragm, respiratory problems will be somewhat alleviated.

When one lies down, nasal congestion sometimes seems to increase. But, upon turning the head to either side, the uppermost nostril may become unblocked or somewhat easier to breathe through. For whatever the reason, a tumbler of Old John Barleycorn will narrow the passageways all the more. A hot meal or coffee may also cause the nose to run, after which the nasal blockage may become more unpleasant. When it rains, the sufferer may experience yet more congestion.

At times like these, my *quickest* (but by no means the only) relief came from the astringent, expectorant, and stimulating action provided by certain nontoxic and non-habit-forming herbal smoking formulas described in the next chapter.

"AIR BLOWING": When undergoing an asthma attack, some have reportedly received relief by vigorously blowing all air possible (a small amount though it may actually be) through a soda straw into a large jar of water in an effort to create a bubbling action in the water.

This unique remedy is said to expand overly tight or spastic airways and allow stale air to escape from the lungs. Another method, which reputedly helps emphysema victims release air from the lungs without rupturing already damaged bronchial air sacs, consists of forcefully exhaling through a small drinking straw (or through nearly closed or pursed lips) as routinely as possible. This exercise has also been recommended for asthmatics. Of course, even a small hernia (or some other organic problem) might prevent certain persons from engaging in these therapies. If you have any tendency to a hernia, check with your doctor before trying these exercises.

Not long ago I read an interesting report by an M.D. who advocates a pursed-lip breathing exercise for his asthma patients. A burning candle is put at mouth level on a table about six inches away. The patient places both hands on his upper abdomen and, as he inhales as deeply as possible, he presses his hands inward on his upper abdomen and blows through pursed or nearly shut lips so as to *bend* the candle flame but *not* extinguish it. This therapy is to be performed once or twice daily for five minutes and the patient is instructed to move back two to four inches each day until he is able to bend the flame from a distance of thirty-six inches.

FIGHTING THE ELEMENTS: Wearing a comfortable hat and warm footgear should prove beneficial to respiratory combatants while outdoors during cold weather. I heard of one sufferer who claimed wondrous results from wearing a ski mask during periods of severe sinus and bronchial attacks. Being warmly clad outdoors is good strategy in cold weather but it is usually wise to go lightly attired indoors.

When summer returns, the hay fever victim may want to purchase a good grade of glare-proof sunglasses to protect or soothe itchy or reddened eyes when exposed to excessive sunlight. The large, curved sunglass designs may partially prevent airborne pollens and dust from blowing into the eyes, but some hay fever fighters have found greater relief by remaining indoors with the windows down on windy days marked by heavy pollen overdrift.

Respiratory troopers of all varieties have occasionally resorted to wearing "unkind weather" masks for walking in the cold, mowing the lawn or dusting, vacuuming, sweeping, or silently rebuking smokers. Even such a small thing as regularly washing the face and hands with warm water during undue pollen "fallout" may possibly aid some hay fever sufferers. But whatever the weather, dusting with somewhat damp cloths (or even covering brooms with damp cloths when sweeping) should prove helpful to anyone tormented by house dust.

RESPIRATORY MANIPULATIONS: While I have had little experience with reflexology or pressure point therapy or massages, there are those who praise such "manipulations." For example, some have allegedly found throat, sinus and bronchial tube relief from thumb massaging both feet regularly under the big toe, along with the nearby area under the three middle toes. A quite energetic, pressing, circular-type motion is advocated and the experimenter (if not, I presume, too weak from laughing) is directed to thoroughly "work out" any tenderness or soreness encountered.

At least one practitioner claims throat and bronchial region consolation from massaging several times daily the same general area of the hands, but he adds that the sufferer should also massage the "webs" between the thumbs and three middle fingers. Another unorthodox notion was related to me by an elderly gentleman. He told me that when his nose appeared ready to "fill up," he prevented blockage by briskly rubbing his ears until they were exceedingly warm. The only thing I obtained from this manipulation was some well-deserved ear soreness but, if it works for you, do it!

As for unblocking the nose during a cold, I never got around to putting thirty-second thumb pressures upon any small "lumps" or "humps" found under one or both armpits. Nor did I ever seriously contemplate relieving clogged sinuses, earaches, headaches, or nausea by applying thumb pressure against the roof of my mouth. However, there just might be something beneficial in the application of hot cloths to the spine during an asthma attack, as well as vigorously massaging the spine in an upward circling motion. In fact, when plagued by congestion miseries, some have gotten relief from heavy phlegm, muscular aches, coughs, and colds by massaging into the chest, back and throat that old standby Vicks VapoRub. (This remedy is *not* to be taken internally or applied inside the nose.) By increasing the flow of blood to the surface of the skin, massaging with Vicks VapoRub (or a similar natural formula) should have a relaxing effect upon the bronchitis sufferer in particular.

Some osteopathic physicians have claimed success in freeing the bronchial tubes of mucus congestion by massaging between the ribs with the tips of the fingers.

PILLOW STUFFING THERAPY: While some respiratory distress has been traced to sleeping on the wrong kind of pillows (feather), early pioneers at times claimed respite from hay fever or asthma woes after sleeping on pillows filled with dried elder leaves. Several species of the herb life everlasting (especially the flowers) were also found helpful. Small pillows crammed with hops (on occasion sprinkled with alcoholic spirits to fetch out the essence) were likewise held worthy in some parts for sleeplessness.

WATER WORKS: Many doctors instruct asthma and bronchitis sufferers to *greatly increase* their water intake (I much prefer bottled apple juice to city water offerings of doubtful purity) and at least one M.D. has written that hay fever patients should increase their fluid intake as well. This therapy is, of course, designed to thin dense mucus secretions and make them more watery so that breathing is less difficult.

As one refrains from unhealthy practices, substitutes sound ones, and a feeling of well-being gradually floods the soul in consequence, there can scarcely be any more sublime words of encouragement in all the English tongue than those that declare: "Amazing grace, how sweet the sound/That saved a wretch like me!/I once was lost, but now am found/Was blind, but now I see." (John Newton, 1779.)

CHAPTER VII

THE HERBAL APPROACH (OR BREWING, CHEWING, INHALING, SNIFFING AND SMOKING HERBS)

And God said, Let the earth bring
forth grass, the herb yielding seed,
and the fruit tree yielding fruit
after his kind, whose seed is in
itself, upon the earth: And it was
so. (Genesis 1:11)

To many students of the Bible, it seems that God intended to bestow on man the means by which a wondrously disease-free existence could be realized by those who reasonably followed His natural health laws. In Genesis 1:31, we note "And God saw everything that He had made, and, behold, it was very good." This does not, of course, mean that *everything* is good to eat but rather that God considered everything He created to be good for humankind (or other life) in some particular way.

For example, belladonna (*Atropa belladonna*, known also as deadly nightshade, is a powerful narcotic. While it is claimed to be a valuable medicinal herb under certain highly controlled circumstances, it is also exceedingly poisonous. Yet there are over 2,000 members of the nightshade family including potatoes, peppers, eggplants, tomatoes and the popular poison tobacco. However, God equipped mankind with a certain intelligence and when He commanded man to subdue the earth, He obviously did not intend for His highest creation to utilize belladonna as a food or to incapacitate the lungs with Lady Nicotine in her many forms.

Let it now be noted that NATURE'S HERBS IMPROPERLY USED CAN BE DETRIMENTAL AND THE USER SHOULD THUS EXERCISE CAUTION AS TO WHICH BOTANICALS ARE UTILIZED—AS WELL AS HOW MUCH. When it comes to natural remedies (as well as "unnatural" ones), be sure you know *what* you're taking and what the possible side effects are.

Following are a few of the most *potentially dangerous* respiratory herbs. DO NOT USE: aconite (monkshood and wolfsbane), bloodroot, cherry laurel (*Prunus laurocerasus*) or cocillana bark, copaiba resin, dropwort (deadtongue, horsebane, or water fennel), grindelia (rosin weed or gum plant), Indian turnip (Jack-in-the-pulpit or any member of the *Arum* family), henbane, jaborandi, larkspur, passion flower (though I have eaten the fruit, called a maypop, with relish on numbers of occasions without dread), pulsatilla, rue (garden or herb-of-grace), and spurge (various *Euphorbia* species). NEVER DRINK "TEAS" MADE FROM SUCH HERBS! (See Bibliography for books on identifying safe and poisonous botanicals).

BREWING AND DRINKING YOUR HERBS

Before discussing the preparation of beneficial herbs, let me emphasize here that herbs tend to work slowly. Because one doesn't think anything is happening during the first several weeks doesn't mean that the natural remedy isn't working. A fair trial period should be allowed.

In herbal language, a DECOCTION involves boiling (or slowly simmering) the herb(s) for from ten to thirty minutes, depending upon obstinacy encountered and final strength desired. Hard roots or seeds, as well as inner and outer barks, are usually prepared as decoctions. Straining is necessary before drinking the resulting tea. In preparing a decoction, some tea drinkers boil or simmer the herb(s) approximately ten minutes and then, cutting off the heat, allow a *steeping* period of even longer duration to obtain a greater botanical "essence." Fresh botanicals of the hard type (roots, barks, seeds with tough coverings) would ordinarily require less boiling or simmering than the dried ones—perhaps half as long.

An INFUSION is different from a decoction because the tea is prepared *without boiling* the herb(s). The ingredients are dropped into *boiling* water and allowed to stand (or steep) until the water cools. As a rule, I cover my infusions with a plastic lid during the steeping process to lessen evaporation. The tea can be rewarmed after straining. Soft materials (dried or fresh) such as flowers, leaves, and seeds not overly hard are normally prepared as infusions. While roots and barks are usually boiled or simmered (see DECOCTION), althaea roots and slippery elm inner bark are so soft in texture that a superior tea may be obtained by the more gentle infusion method. Although directions on the herbal tea boxes sold in health food centers generally recommend a steeping time of three to five minutes, I usually allow my infusions to stand for approximately ten minutes. I have sometimes permitted them to remain as much as one-half hour when a stronger drink is needed. I strongly recommend that the respiratory sufferer add a teaspoon or two of raw honey and some lemon juice (to taste) to each eight-ounce cup of herb tea. Always be sure to wash thoroughly any natural products before brewing (or chewing).

REMINDERS: Children should, naturally, be given only half or less of what would be the adult dose of herb tea.

Do not take herbs and drugs at the same time because they do not usually work well together. Of course, the gradual and sensible use of herbal teas (along with proper nutrition and the rest of my program) should aid in the eventual eliminations of respiratory drugs for many people.

Drinkers of herb tea might wish to invest (for a small sum) in one of the small globe-shaped, stainless steel strainers. The herb(s) can be placed inside this easily opened and closed contraption and securely dropped into a cup of boiling water for steeping without any messiness whatever.

A SELECTION OF HERBS FOR TEA

The following herbs were chosen for their beneficial effects on respiratory complaints. I also believe they produce teas that are among the safest of those made from any botanicals.

Althaea or marsh mallow (*Althaea officinalis*): ASTHMA and BRONCHITIS. For what is widely hailed as a relaxing, diuretic and soothing respiratory tea, drop one teaspoonful of althaea's quite soft roots into one cup of boiling water and steep for about ten minutes. Similar results have also been claimed by steeping two tablespoons of the flowers and leaves in one cup of steaming water for about seven minutes before straining. The root tea is generally favored but whatever the part(s) used, drink one cup daily with raw honey.

Anise or aniseed *(Pimpinella anisum)*: BRONCHITIS. A teaspoon of the soft seeds of this aromatic herb can be dropped into a cup of boiling water for about ten minutes, strained, and freely consumed "as is" for not only the "dry" cough of bronchitis but for acidity, insomnia (often with hot milk), nausea, digestive gases or upsets. For hoarseness, put four ounces of anise seeds in approximately ten ounces of water, boil for fifteen to twenty minutes, mash all the water possible out while straining, and add one-fourth to one-third cup of honey and a tablespoon of brandy or cherry vodka. This remedy may be taken at the rate of one tablespoonful every half-hour of the day. Herbalists believe aniseed to be tonic, stimulative, carminative, expectorant and, to some degree, antispasmodic. Anise has a peculiar sweetness all its own and some users enjoy the tea without honey.

Catnip or catmint *(Nepeta cataria)*: BRONCHITIS. A teaspoonful of the aromatic whole herb can be dropped in a cup of boiling water and allowed to stand for about ten minutes before straining and flavoring with honey to alleviate chronic bronchitis, colds, restlessness, an unsettled or acid stomach, intestinal griping, and, to some degree, a nervous headache. While several cups of catnip tea can be consumed daily, large amounts of the warm or hot tea may possibly have an emetic effect. In earlier times, catnip was considered helpful for colds when used in hot foot baths. (Cats are strangely drawn to this herb because of a fascination with the odor and will often uproot any unprotected catnip discovered during their prowlings.)

Coltsfoot (*Tussilago farfara*): ASTHMA, BRONCHITIS and HAY FEVER. Widely acclaimed as an astringent, an expectorant and as being soothing to inflamed parts, coltsfoot appears beneficial for sinusitis and all sorts of respiratory problems, including the so-called "dry cough" of bronchitis with, in some instances, its attendant feverishness. Steep one to three teaspoons of the leaves (or flowers if available) in a cup of boiling water for twenty to thirty minutes before straining. Rewarm and take one cupful daily with raw honey. Hay fever sufferers have reportedly steeped a teaspoonful each of coltsfoot, mullein leaves and wild plum inner bark for about thirty minutes in a pint of boiling water. After straining, this infusion was taken two or three times daily at the rate of four tablespoons per dose. Coltsfoot also appears to work particularly well mingled with althaea roots and horehound, sweetened with honey, for asthma and bronchitis woes.

Comfrey (*Symphytum officinale*): ASTHMA, BRONCHITIS and HAY FEVER. This herb, with its astringent, demulcent, and expectorant properties, is claimed beneficial for digestive system problems, "tickling" coughs, sundry internal ulcers, liver complaints, and bloody urine. In fact, many pioneer herb users regarded comfrey as about the closest thing to a "cure-all" known, and it has a long record of being used (internally and externally) when all else falls short. To prepare a tea, simmer one or two teaspoons of the mucilaginous root in a cup and one-half of water for around ten minutes. Drink the resulting tea hot and well fortified with raw honey and a few squirts of fresh lemon juice for superior results. Or several tablespoons of the leaves can be dropped into a cup of boiling water and steeped for about ten minutes before straining. Whatever the part(s) used, drink one or two cups daily. Several teaspoons of comfrey roots can be boiled in two cups of water for about twenty minutes and used as a gargle to relieve some throat irritations or hoarseness. For respiratory ailments, comfrey leaves are not as highly commended as the roots. However, the demulcent herbs, of which comfrey is a leading example, are believed soothing to the body's mucous membranes. Other demulcent herbs with respiratory properties are althaea (any part), barley, coltsfoot leaves, fenugreek seeds, figs, flaxseeds (*mature* seeds *only* since the immature seed pods are toxic), ginseng roots, licorice roots, olive oil, mullein and plantain (roots or flowers more than leaves) and slippery elm inner bark.

A word of warning here: An Australian scientist has shown that comfrey contains one of a group of four or five toxic alkaloids suspected of being or known to be carcinogens. Dr. Claude Culvenor of the Animal Health

Division of the Australian Commonwealth Scientific and Industrial Research Organization said, "It is probable that the type [of alkaloid] found in comfrey is also carcinogenic. While it is unlikely that anybody eating comfrey in *small quantities* would suffer serious effects, its regular use as a *green vegetable* could cause chronic liver damage or worse. Plants in the same family have caused human poisonings in the USSR, Africa, India and Afganistan after their accidental consumption in bread over a period of one or two years. The evidence of these outbreaks, considering the amount of the alkaloid we have measured in comfrey, *suggests* that daily consumption of several young leaves of the plant over a similarly lengthy period will lead to serious disease."

Although more research must be done to determine comfrey's *possible* side effects, cautious readers may wish to abstain from the use of this plant. As with all things in life, the benefits must be weighed against the possible detriments.

Elecampane (*Inula helenium*): ASTHMA, BRONCHITIS and HAY FEVER. There have long been reports that elecampane roots are antiseptic, astringent, diuretic and expectorant; have special worth as a stomach conditioner, digestive system stimulant, expellant of kidney or bladder stones on occasion and reliever of blocked or sluggish urine. Whatever the truth, simmer a teaspoonful of the rootstock for ten minutes or thereabouts in sufficient water to retain one cupful for gradual sipping during the day. Both honey and lemon juice may be added. Elecampane is not infrequently combined with such respiratory herbs as comfrey roots, horehound blossoms, or wild cherry inner bark, and syrups, as well as cough lozenges made from elecampane roots, graced the marketplace in other times.

Fenugreek (*Trigonella foenumgraecum*): BRONCHITIS. Slowly simmer several teaspoons of the highly mucilaginous seeds for about ten minutes in enough water to retain a full cup upon straining. Drink several cups daily (sufficiently bolstered with raw honey and possibly lemon juice to mask the bitter taste) for not only bronchitis and any attendant fever but inflammations of the intestinal tract and stomach. Moreover, if early claims are to be believed, gargling with fenugreek tea may relieve a sore throat. This is a very ancient herb with a proven value to mankind and it is still highly esteemed in the Orient.

Ginseng (*Panax quinquefolium*): BRONCHITIS and possibly ASTHMA. On occasion, a cup of hot ginseng tea seems to open blocked sinuses somewhat. Nonetheless, it is difficult to ignore the awe-inspiring claims that have surrounded this herb since long before Christ. It has been celebrated by the Chinese and others as a near "cure-all" with virtues well beyond the ordinary. If used regularly, ginseng root tea is said to be beneficial for sundry chest problems, including consumption and emphysema; the common cold; feverishness; poor appetite; nausea; stomach miseries; urinary tract or other inflammations; various glandular disorders; nervous system complaints; headaches; constipation; hiccoughs; hemor-rhagings; sciatica; and spots before the eyes. A little of the dried root can be simmered in sufficient water to produce a cupful of tea but, unfortunately, good roots-tock is becoming both more costly and progressively harder to find. In fact, the day may not be far removed when ginseng is declared an endangered species in North Carolina since an estimated 1,500 commercial dig-gers, largely mountain folk, were gathering ginseng dur-ing 1977 alone. The ground rootstock, when obtainable, can be quickly prepared as an infusion and very little of the powder is required. There appears to be no known toxicity from drinking several cups daily when one can afford it, and I have heard that some Chinese doctors advocate one cupful per day as an overall health booster.

Horehound (*Marrubium vulgare*): ASTHMA and BRONCHITIS. This herb has known commercial popu-larity for its use in beverages, old-fashioned candies, and throat lozenges taken for chronic coughs, hoarseness or catarrh. A pint of boiling water is usually poured over an ounce of horehound (whole herb) and allowed to stand about ten minutes before straining. It appears best to slowly sip a half cup of the tea per sitting, three or four times daily, flavored with ample honey after reheat-ing. Lemon juice reputedly improves the respiratory ac-tion on occasion. In early times, some victims of hoarse-ness advocated dropping an ounce of horehound into a pint of boiling water for two hours before straining and drinking four teaspoons per dose several times daily. Infusions of horehound, doctored with cayenne pepper, were also taken for coughing spells. Horehound is generally regarded as a tonic herb with aromatic, stimulative, diuretic and expectorant virtues.

Licorice (*Glycyrrhiza glabra*): ASTHMA and BRONCHITIS. The root of this somewhat laxative, diuretic, thirst-quenching, demulcent, and expectorant herb was possibly known to the ancient Sumerians prior to reaching Egypt. Indeed, licorice was reportedly used at least three centuries before Christ for the "dry cough" and hoarseness. Not only is it still taken in some quarters for general chest complaints but is claimed of benefit for peptic ulcers as well as kidney, bladder and stomach ailments. The average intake appears to be one cup daily prepared by boiling one teaspoonful of the root in sufficient water for ten minutes or by *steeping* the same, until fairly strong, *after* the water has been allowed to boil. If used for the so-called "dry cough" of bronchitis, it may be best to drink the tea as hot as can be tolerated and fortified with raw honey, although licorice has its own peculiar sweetness and there are many who use no honey at all in it.

Now, according to Frank A. Finnerty, M.D., consuming a "lot" of licorice candy regularly can raise the blood pressure in some patients. He also reports that an ulcer treatment medicine containing several of the same basic chemicals as licorice can produce the same reaction in such individuals. One particular candy addict, who reportedly ate a pound of licorice weekly, had a blood pressure reading of 170/120 which dropped to 140/92 within three months after being denied licorice. There are other medical reports that the consumption of hoglike amounts of licorice candy while taking digitalis-type heart drugs may possibly cause adverse reactions. Headache sufferers have also been warned against becoming licorice loonies. I mention all of this in passing for what it is worth. If I should crave a cup of licorice tea, I'd have no more fear of it than those over-the-counter preparations containing therapeutic amounts of licorice. Also, licorice has historically been considered as soothing to the mucous membranes and certain herbalists advocate mingling it with figs to relieve asthma.

Mullein, Aaron's rod, great mullein (*Verbascum thapsus*): ASTHMA, BRONCHITIS and HAY FEVER. Among other names, this widespread herb is called Indian tobacco in a number of localities. It is interesting to note that an unrelated plant, the potentially poisonous lobelia (or vomitroot), is also known as Indian tobacco. While the antispasmodic, astringent, demulcent, expectorant, diuretic and slightly nervine leaves of mullein are commonly used, it is said that an infusion of the flowers not only soothes the mucous membranes but will alleviate chest aches and encourage sleep. The same claims, however, are made for the leaves used alone and mullein leaf tea has for generations been acclaimed beneficial for the croup, sinusitis, bleeding in the lungs, colds, hoarseness, tuberculosis, general inflammations and dropsy, in addition to asthma, bronchitis and hay fever complaints. It is also said that public speakers or singers can somewhat control their voice problems by regularly drinking or gargling mullein tea. I find this plant thriving along railroad tracks but have to harvest it before the track maintenance crews spray it with insecticides. One or two cupfuls, prepared by steeping at least a teaspoon of the leaves (or flowers) in a cup of boiling water for ten minutes before straining, can be consumed daily, supplemented with raw honey. For asthmatic coughs, a strong tea was reportedly brewed by early settlers from the "root bark" (outer covering peeled from the root) of common (or great) mullein and given to children at frequent intervals (sweetened to a syrupy consistency with honey) at the rate of four teaspoons per dose.

Plantain (*Plantago major, lanceolata, etc.*): BRONCHITIS and HAY FEVER. All parts (exclusive of the seeds, unless one desires a laxative condition) can be used. Prepare a tea by dropping at least a tablespoonful of the dried herb in a cup of boiling water and steeping about ten minutes prior to straining and flavoring with raw honey. Two cups daily can, I believe, be consumed with gain by some sufferers. However, in years past, I frequently ate a few freshly picked plantain (or mullein) leaves and obtained some antihistamine action for hay fever attacks, particularly when supplemented with Vitamin C (in lesser amounts of this vitamin than would ordinarily be needed). Plantain is considered astringent, expectorant, alterative, (agent that can change or alter unhealthy physical conditions and restore normal functions), demulcent, diuretic and somewhat tonic. In addition to bronchitis, hay fever, colds and sinusitis, early settlers used plantain tea with regularity for such diverse infirmities as kidney or bladder complaints, neuralgia, bed-wetting, worms (stomach and intestinal), ulcers, lumbar pains, diarrhea, piles and some blood disorders. Moreover, a number of old time herbalists believed plantain poultices would control rattlesnake and mad dog bites!

Saw palmetto (*Serenoa serrulata*): ASTHMA, BRONCHITIS and possibly HAY FEVER. This southern coastal palm produces a berry (actually the mixtures I've purchased were mostly berry husks rather than the hard, crushed or ground berries) claimed not only beneficial for the aforesaid complaints but for whooping cough, tuberculosis, sore throat, digestive disorders, Bright's disease and all glandular affections (including swollen or aching testes and prostatitis). When one ounce of dried berries is fully pulverized into powder and steeped ten minutes in one pint of boiling water, one teaspoonful may be taken three times daily. However, if one prefers to steep one teaspoon of the rather soft berry husks in a cup of boiling water, one may drink one or two cups per day. Saw palmetto berries appear to be astringent, expectorant, diuretic, tonic, and to some degree antiseptic, sedative and stimulative in action. Additionally, this herb allegedly possesses nutritive properties capable of not only rebuilding glandular tissues but adding weight and strength to muscles that have deteriorated for one reason or another. The husks come close to being the best single respiratory smoking ingredient I've ever found.

Slippery elm (*Ulmus fulva*): BRONCHITIS. While the mucilaginous inner bark of slippery elm has been much heralded for bronchitis, it is rarely mentioned as a specific for asthma. However, the fact that slippery elm has demulcent, expectorant and nutritive properties should certainly make it of some worth to asthmatics. At any rate, tea brewed from the inner bark has long been used as a homemade balm for chronic coughs associated with bronchitis, as a gargle for less complicated throat irritations, and as a soothing agent for inflamed mucous membranes of the lungs, intestinal tract, kidneys and stomach. It is said that the stomach can abide slippery elm tea when other liquids are less than gentle. The brew may be flavored with raw honey, cinnamon or lemon juice to one's taste. I have made a fairly acceptable chest remedy by dissolving slippery elm throat lozenges (from the health food store) in a cup of boiling water for sipping. There have even been claims that bleeding of the lungs has been stayed by the regular use of this botanical. Whatever the truth, an ounce of slippery elm inner bark can be steeped for an hour or more in a pint of boiling water, strained, reheated, flavored to taste, and taken by the teaspoonful several times during the course of an hour for inflamed mucous membranes. Two teaspoons of the inner bark can also be steeped in a cup of boiling water for about an hour, simmered before straining, flavored with honey, and several cups consumed during the day as necessary. (Teas derived from powdered inner bark require far less steeping time and, of course, about one-half as much of the concentrated powder is needed.)

CAUTION: For one reason or another, herbs not used for tea include: agrimony (cocklebur), angelica, blue vervain, boneset, borage, improperly identified dwarf or stinging nettle species, garden thyme, hyssop (Hyssopus officinalis), parsley, sage (Salvia officinalis), American spikenard, wood betony, and yerba santa among others.

A leaf infusion of agrimony appears primarily used as a gargel for mouth or throat irritations. There seems much confusion as to the average intake of American spikenard, angelica, blue vervain and wood betony. Boneset (*Eupatorium perfoliatum*) is apparently best taken three to six times daily, unheated, by the *teaspoonful*, rather than by the cupful. Extended or excessive use of borage, hyssop, garden thyme or sage can cause toxic symptoms. Parsley should be avoided in the presence of inflamed kidneys. Stinging nettle or its cousin dwarf nettle (*Urtica species*) may be mistaken for several unrelated plants of toxic nature that are also called "nettle" locally (which is why I always purchased imported nettle for testing). Yerba santa (holy herb) may contain traces of the toxic phenol.

Be sure you obtain your herbs from a reliable source. I have been fortunate in the procurement of my herbs. Chuck Snyder, proprietor, Garden of Eden, Inc., 423

Woodburn Road, Cameron Village, Raleigh, North Carolina 27605, has kept me steadily supplied with nontoxic, hard-to-get botanicals for my research for many years. Chuck's establishment has been a godsend to many herbal tea lovers in surrounding areas and talking with Chuck is an experience in itself!

CHEWING (OR EATING) YOUR HERBS

Certain carefully selected herbs with beneficial respiratory properties can be chewed outright or eaten raw in salads. Even the best commercial methods known for preparing foods destroy, alter or weaken vital ingredients that remain comparatively undisturbed in fresh or properly dried herbs. As a rule, approximately one and one-half to two times as much of the fresh herbs are used as the concentrated dried ones. Of course, be sure to wash any leaves, roots or bark before chewing or eating.

Among the herbs with respiratory properties that can be utilized as flavoring agents in salads are almonds (demulcent), anise seeds (expectorant, stimulative), celery seeds (sedative or nervine), basil or sweet basil (antispasmodic), crushed barley seeds (demulcent), caraway seeds (antispasmodic, somewhat expectorant), crushed cubeb or Java pepper berries (antiseptic, expectorant, stimulative), dill seeds (antispasmodic, calmative), fennel seeds (antispasmodic, expectorant, stimulative), garden radishes (antispasmodic, astringent, but not advised in case of intestinal irritations or stomach problems), garlic cloves (antiseptic, antispasmodic, expectorant), marjoram (antispasmodic, calmative, expectorant), onions (antiseptic, antispasmodic, expectorant), oregano (see marjoram above, of which oregano is a "wild" species similarly used), savory (astringent, expectorant, stimulative, the tea of which is of some value as a gargle for sore throat), sweet or lemon balm (antispasmodic, calmative), and sunflower seeds (expectorant).

These "respiratory salad herbs" range in flavor from the bitterness of celery seeds (a fairly good salt substitute) to the licoricelike sweetness of anise or fennel seeds and the mildness of sunflower seeds. While not listed in this grouping, I feel that sesame seeds used in salads regularly may have a soothing (demulcent) effect on irritated mucous membranes. Of course, herbs such as celery seed must be used sparingly because a small amount will go a long way tastewise. If a problem of palatability arises, one can pit the aromatic, spicy or fragrant qualities of some herbs against the bitterness of others.

While I would not hesitate to use hyssop (*Hyssopus officinalis*), garden sage (*Salvia officinalis*) or garden thyme (*Thymus vulgaris*) as herbal smoking ingredients, I would (pending further research) hesitate to consume them with regularity as teas or in salads since their excessive or prolonged use may possibly cause toxic symptoms. For example, it is said that thyme taken in excess can overactivate the thyroid gland or trigger digestive upsets in some individuals. Of course, thyme has a history of being used in cough remedies or as a muscle relaxant and it is widely employed as a flavoring agent for meats and soups. The intake of the medicinal ingredient thymol, which is derived from thyme (as well as origanum oil or lavender oil), is said to be only .067 grams. Of course, many herbs or foods that are generally considered safe when consumed in a normal manner contain *substances* that can be harmful or even deadly if *extracted* and consumed without medical supervision in the *concentrated* or essential oil form.

CHEWABLE HERBS

Althaea or marsh mallow: A teaspoonful of the remarkably soft rootstock can be slowly chewed until all the juice has been swallowed, after which the pulp is discarded. This should be of gradual aid to asthma or bronchitis sufferers when there is insufficient time to brew a tea. There are also claims that althaea roots are soothing to stomach ulcers. On one occasion, chewing some althaea roots (in company with several calcium tablets) seemed to momentarily soothe the ache in an accidentally cracked rear tooth until I could reach the dentist. Dabbing the area with oil of cloves might have worked better but I mention this for what it is worth.

Anise or aniseed: On a day with digestive upsets, any number of individuals will probably chew anise seeds and experience the "blessed relief" credited to the antacids glorified in the ads. Also, anyone suffering from the so-called "dry cough" of bronchitis may want to regularly chew anise seeds long enough to test their efficacy, if any, in this particular regard. Apart from these considerations, the pleasant and licoricelike flavor of anise seeds should endear them to many.

Cloves: When annoyed by a tickling sensation in the throat, early settlers reportedly chewed several cloves. Chewing cloves may also, on occasion, alleviate sneezing during a hay fever attack for certain individuals.

Coltsfoot: It may be possible that some asthma, bronchitis or hay fever sufferers can beneficially chew a teaspoon of coltsfoot leaves each day in lieu of a cupful of tea.

Comfrey: Several tablespoonfuls of the leaves may be regularly tested for asthma, bronchitis or hay fever instead of the tea. While it is only hearsay, there have been reports that several asthmatics have been "cured" by regularly consuming comfrey leaves fresh from the garden. However, I cannot resist believing there is much more to overcoming asthma than this, especially if the condition is solidly established. Aside from aiding respiratory ailments, the considerable mucilage found in comfrey (don't overlook the possible value of okra either) may be of benefit in maintaining good elimination.*

Cubeb berries (Java pepper): These antiseptic berries smell very spicy and have a more or less sharp and bitter taste that produces a curious "coolness" in the mouth suggestive of peppermint. Cubeb berries are not to be confused with dried peppercorns or black pepper ber-

---

* Please see pages 152-3 for recent warning concerning alleged misuse of comfrey.

ries. They are likely to appear on the spice racks as Java pepper rather than cubebs. In some instances, our frontier ancestors successfully chewed unripe (but dried) cubebs to alleviate uncomplicated sore throats. Cubeb berries undoubtedly enjoyed their greatest commercial fame when crushed and combined in sufficient measure with smoking tobacco to combat "smoker's hack," coughs and catarrh.

Fennel: As much as three teaspoons of the licorice-dill-flavored seeds have been steeped in a cup of boiling water for about ten minutes, strained, and sipped for relief of gas, acidity, abdominal cramps, mucus congestion, and sluggish appetite. Some consider the tea effective as a gargle against hoarseness or cough. However, chewing the seeds outright may be of some merit against bronchial congestion, particularly if mingled with honey. Fennel is more palatable if chewed in combination with aniseed.

Garlic: Since time unknown, garlic cloves have been chewed for asthma, bronchitis, and colds, often in league with honey, and there are various claims that parsley roots, fennel seeds and even hot chocolate have some ability to neutralize the rankness. Garlic capsules fortified with parsley are sold in health food stores. These are supposed to retain the many therapeutic values of garlic without allowing the sometimes horrifying odor from seeping through the pores.

Ginger: Ginger root is often chewed "as is" for a cough or sore throat and discarded after the juice is spent. By the time ginger roots reach the supermarket, however, they may be too hard for chewing by the average person.

Ginseng: Southern mountaineers have claimed that chewing ginseng (often called "sang" in their picturesque speech) will strengthen a weak stomach, aid indigestion and alleviate tickling sensations in the throat. Ginseng has recently sold for $105 a pound and has now been placed on the list of endangered species in Georgia. Under such conditions as these, chewing ginseng roots could well become a lost art. The cultivation of ginseng is said to be exceedingly difficult and the medicinal virtues of the wild plants are superior to domestic offerings.

Horehound: Try chewing this bitter, tonic herb in combination with honey or aniseed for relief of respiratory imperfections, particularly throat huskiness and the common cough. (Note: Horehound, in its "refined extract state" is well represented in commercial cough drops.)

Leek: The imaginative respiratory sufferer can chew the antispasmodic leek regularly, perhaps, instead of its stronger brother garlic, for the gradual control of bronchial congestion. Of course, sampling honey while chewing upon leeks, etc., is advisable.

Licorice: The extracted juice of licorice roots is much used by the pharmaceutical industry in cough drops or throat lozenges. Chewing a little licorice root thoroughly before discarding it should achieve similar results, particularly if supplemented with lemon juice, honey and a little ground capsicum (cayenne or red pepper), for good measure, if available.

Mullein: In the struggling days before my hay fever was brought well under control, I gathered the large velvetlike mullein leaves and sometimes regularly chewed several tablespoonsfuls *fresh* (less *dried* herb is needed) each day instead of making a tea. I found that, directly after chewing the fresh mullein (well washed to remove any possible grittiness), supplementation with Vitamin C (in particular), B2, B6, pantothenic acid and honey controlled the hay fever even better. (At the time, I didn't realize *smoking* dried mullein produced quicker results than almost anything else if a pollen fallout emergency came to pass.)

Onion: Consider chewing this herb for respiratory ailments on a regular basis. Bronchitis and emphysema are reportedly aided by nucleic acid (or RNA) in onions.

Plantain: I believe that chewing several fresh plantain leaves (*Plantago species*), particularly if followed with Vitamin C, B2, B6, pantothenic acid and honey, will prove of some value to some hay fever fighters.

Slippery elm: The inner bark of this soothing herb can be chewed quite frequently (discarding the pulp after the juice is fully removed) for ordinary coughs and throat irritations. (Frontier herbalists wrote that the inner bark would even sustain life for a considerable time if all other provender grew scarce.)

Coordinating one's chewings (and brewings!) with well-chosen mineral-vitamin supplements may produce better results in the campaign against respiratory problems. In chewing herbs, anise seeds appear superior to all others when chewed in combination with less tasty ones.

The chewing of UNDYED, especially prepared citrus peelings twice daily was suggested earlier. However, there has been ongoing controversy as to the toxicity of dyes used on fruits. Recently Citrus Red No. 2 Monoazo was cited as potentially toxic if consumed in quantity. In addition to monoazo (composed of diazonium and the potentially toxic phenol), this dye contains a 2-naphthol constituent that has been condemned also as harmful in quantity. Unless, therefore, one can obtain naturally grown UNDYED citrus, it may be the better part of wisdom to eat the fruit only and forgo chewing the peelings.

On rare occasions, one may discover a little grittiness in chewing herbs not properly cleaned before drying. To avoid this, gently stir the herbs selected for therapeutic chewing (particularly the leafy ones) in a little bowl of cool water until thoroughly cleansed.

INHALING AND SNIFFING HERBS

Inhaling certain herbal vapors can help unblock stuffy passageways. But it is best to inhale the vapors for only a few minutes at a time and not run any risk of exerting oneself. Herbal inhalation therapy is simple. Stand near a pot of heated water with a towel held in tent fashion over the head and cautiously inhale the herbal vapors. Use a small amount of eucalyptus leaves, peppermint, spearmint, yellow poplar or tulip tree buds, balsam poplar buds, aniseed, lavender flowers, cloves, birch leaves, cinnamon bark, raw onions, linden flowers, benzoin gum, sage, powdered ginger, mullein roots, horehound, or catnip. Some experimentation may be needed to determine the actual amount of water and herb(s) required for the best results, but generally a teaspoon of the unrefined herb will be adequate.

Instead of inhaling the vapors of these herbs in their unrefined states, it is perhaps more convenient to go to the druggist and buy one's oil of eucalyptus, tincture of benzoin compound, Vicks VapoRub Decongestant Ointment (for use in a steam vaporizer) and oil of peppermint. USE THESE HERBAL INHALATION PREPARATIONS ONLY AS DIRECTED as they are in their *concentrated* forms and the labels warn against any possible misuse. I was surprised to learn that the label on one brand of eucalyptus oil directs the user to "Put a *few drops* in boiling water and inhale the vapors," whereas the label on another brand reads "Pour *one teaspoon* into a pint of boiling water and inhale the vapors. May be repeated three times daily." Obviously there is a wide range in the dosage between the two brands. Both labels instruct the buyer to seek professional assistance or contact a poison control center promptly if the oil is accidentally ingested because doses as small as a single gram of the *highly concentrated product* have induced coma and as little as 3.5 grams have proven fatal.

Menthol, which is obtained largely from peppermint oil, is also used in inhalation formulas. While it is not as potent as oil of eucalyptus, it can cause digestive upsets or coma if it is not used as the label directs. Properly used, oils of eucalyptus and peppermint are of great value in respiratory medicines from cough drops to inhalants. (This opinion does not include such inhalant substances as epinephrine, Isoproterenol or the cortisone-type ingredients.) Of course, the best thing about buying laboratory-prepared herbal inhalants such as eucalyptus, peppermint or benzoin is the fact that they have been scientifically tested as to the proper dosage and, if properly used, the likelihood of any adverse effects would appear small.

Few inhalant substances rival the fame of tincture of benzoin as having expectorant properties. Many a mother with a croupy child, plagued with an unproductive cough or chronic congestion, has sung the praises of this herb without reservations. The renowned remedy of old, Friar's Balsam, was chiefly derived from tincture of benzoin. Recently I noted the following directions on a bottle of tincture of benzoin compound:

As an inhalant add *one* teaspoonful to a *quart* of *hot* water and inhale the vapors. Use a similar quantity when using mechanical vaporizers. Warning: Persons with a high fever or persistent cough, should not use this product unless directed by a physician. If cough or throat irritation persists, be sure to consult your physician. Ingredients: Fluid extract benzoin compound and alcohol. Warning: In case of accidental ingestion seek professional assistance or contact a poison control center immediately.

Webster's *New World Dictionary* defines benzoin as "A balsamic resin obtained from certain Asiatic trees (genus *Styrax*) and used in medicines and perfumery and as incense." While benzoic acid is derived from gum benzoin, it is also found naturally in anise seeds, wild cherry bark, raspberries, cinnamon, and tea. However, it should be noted that the above brand of tincture of benzoin instructs *one* teaspoonful to a *quart* of *hot* water, whereas Lilly's Tincture No. 10 says on the label: "Tincture benzoin. For steam inhalation. Add *one* teaspoonful to a *pint* of *boiling* water. Contents alcohol 79 percent." Here again the instructions differ and the user should be governed accordingly.

Such ingredients as oil of pine, spirits of camphor, or gum spirits of turpentine are featured in commercial inhalant formulas in very small amounts. Of course, pine resins are the chief source of turpentine or pine oil and a dose of only 15 grams of pure turpentine when taken internally has killed children. A not uncommon label on gum spirits of turpentine reads: "Harmful or fatal if swallowed." While some asthmatics have inhaled vapors derived from boiling pine needles and cones in water several times daily, fighting asthma in this manner may result in too much turpentine reaching the vital organs. Therefore, why should unnecessary risks be taken? Some of the herbal inhalation formulas sold appear to contain potentially risky oils, spirits or extracts, so use these preparations with caution and be sure to follow the label directions.

As for itchy eyes caused by hay fever, one of the best inhalation formulas I ever devised is composed of several teaspoons of the herb peppermint and a teaspoonful of anise seeds boiled in about a pint and one-half of water. The vapors are then inhaled briefly. A little while following the expectorant workings of the herbs, a true astringent action sets in and restrains, to some degree, a "runny" nose. Furthermore, when suffering from nasal stuffiness or tightness-in-the-chest problems, gently inhaling the fumes with the mouth wide open (or directly through the stuffy nose to the extent possible) often gives me a measure of respite. Apparently a nontoxic amount of menthol present in the rising steam was largely responsible for the "cooling" and decongestant action experienced. *NOTE*: Turn the heat completely off and let the vapors *die down* before inhaling *directly through the mouth.* As will be observed with a little experimentation, open-mouth inhalations standing directly near a pot of steadily boiling water can approach the impossible and can constitute a hazard as well.

For treating head colds and nasal stuffiness, there is a rather interesting herbal-based product called Vapex Inhalant. According to the label, it contains "An aromatic mixture of menthol, oils of lavender and eucalyptus, cineole, linalyl acetate, oil of pine, terebene, borneol, alcohol 69 percent." Cineole comes from many essential oils including eucalyptus; linalyl acetate is found naturally in citrus peels, basil, lavender oil, lemon oil, and jasmine oil; terebene is derived from oil of turpentine; and borneol is a kind of camphor that closely resembles true camphor, being found naturally in ginger oil, rosemary, thyme, strawberries, coriander, and nutmeg. However, the label on Vapex Inhalant continues with the following directions: "Apply a few drops of Vapex to the center of a folded handkerchief. Hold handkerchief over your nose and breathe in vapors deeply and frequently." Had I known about this product during the months when I was *gradually* withdrawing from asthma and hay fever tablets, I would have considered substituting it to the extent possible for stronger medicines. If it can be safely used for nasal stuffiness as the label indicates, it may be worth investigating as a partial aid to that specific condition.

In bygone days, doctors reportedly advised patients to boil leeks in water and inhale the vapors in cases of enlarged tonsils. Pomegranate juice and honey were also reportedly "instilled" in the nasal passages to "prevent polyps," but I know of no claims that herbal inhalations will dissolve or prevent this evil.

Some respiratory sufferers may desire to test an automatic "hot steam" vaporizer of the sort sold in many drug stores. A famous herbal preparation, Vicks VapoRub, is put into the "medicine cup" of this type of vaporizer and the steam inhaled for nasal stuffiness (up to eight hours of relief claimed), bronchial mucus congestion, croupy night coughs, laryngitis and huskiness due to colds. The active ingredients in this formula are camphor, menthol, spirits of turpentine, eucalyptus oil, cedar leaf oil, myristica oil and thymol, presumably in sane amounts. A warning on the label reads: "For external application and use in steam only. Do not swallow or place in nostrils." The Vicks people also have another herbally grounded inhalant called Vicks VapoSteam for use in a hot steam vaporizer, wash basin or ordinary bowl. This preparation contains such old-fasioned ingredients as: "Eucalyptus oil, camphor and menthol 12.4 percent. Tincture of benzoin 5 percent. Alcohol 55 percent."

Some people have reportedly inhaled medicinal fumes while comfortably lying on the floor next to a hot steam vaporizer with a sheet covering an oversized umbrella placed near the head. According to some medical reports, many asthma, bronchitis and hay fever sufferers sleep more comfortably by placing an automatic medicinal vaporizer on a table or chair near the bed and gently inhaling the fumes throughout the night. If desired, the sufferer can spend thirty or forty minutes under the umbrella apparatus noted above prior to retiring for the night.

Hay fever was said to have been alleviated for some in earlier days by inhaling fumes derived from scattering coffee grounds over hot coals. The leaves of stinging nettle (*Urtica urens* or related species *only*), as well as mullein roots, were also dried and later burned for inhalation by asthma sufferers in isolated instances. There must, however, be better ways!

Perhaps "sniffing" or "snuffing" certain herbal solutions or "teas" up first one side of the nose and then the other can ease stuffiness for some. Astringent herbs shrink tissues and reduce secretions or discharges such as phlegm. The hay fever combatant may consider making "sniffers" (directions follow) out of the following herbs regarded as astringents: birch leaves or bark, blackberry roots or leaves, coltsfoot leaves, comfrey (any part), life everlasting flowers (*Gnaphalium polycephalum*), goldenrod flowers or leaves, hibiscus flowers (many species), laurel or bay laurel (the same as one finds on the grocery shelves and *not* to be confused with the poisonous mountain laurel), mullein, plantain, saw palmetto berries, savory or summer savory (whole herb), slippery elm inner bark and white oak bark.

During my "sniffing" days, I usually boiled or steeped one or two teaspoons of each herb (or herbs) selected in a pint of water until a fairly good strength was reached. After thoroughly straining and allowing the "tea" to cool sufficiently, I poured it into a "cupped" hand and patiently sniffed it up one nasal passage at a time in an effort to reduce as much swelling as possible. Sometimes I made enough of the solution for three or four sniffing sessions per day. Lemons (and limes) have certain astringent properties and a little fresh lemon juice squeezed into cool water and sniffed gently up the nasal passages several times daily may, if done on a regular basis, help shrink swollen mucous membranes in sinus or hay fever victims. (Some asthmatics or bronchitics have acquired a measure of relief simply by swallowing a tablespoon of lemon juice approximately an hour before each meal-time. Even better results have been attributed to taking a tablespoonful every fifteen minutes throughout the day!) Other herbs with astringent properties that might be used for a "sniffing tea" are cloves, common commercial cinnamon, elecampane roots, raspberry leaves, skullcap (somewhat mild), wild cherry inner bark, and wild plum inner bark.

Another interesting astringent herb is the wax myrtle or bayberry shrub (*Myrica cerifera*). The leaves, bark and even the wax from the fruit have all been boiled at the rate of one teaspoon per eight-ounce cup of water and one or two cups of the tea taken daily for such diverse conditions as diarrhea, scrofula, hemorrhages, jaundice and sore throat (in gargle fashion). The bark seems most praised and some have reportedly sniffed solutions up the nostrils with success for hay fever. But, most astonishingly, nasal stuffiness was once "treated" by using powdered bayberry (presumably the bark) as a snuff in the same manner employed by frontier Americans who snorted or "snuffed" pulverized tobacco (better known as snuff) up the nostrils instead of taking it as a "dip" by way of the mouth!

Seemingly, herbs that are demulcent in action (soothing to inflamed parts), as well as astringent, would be the better "sniffers" when nasal soreness is most manifest. Noteworthy botanicals in this category are coltsfoot, comfrey, mullein, plantain and slippery elm. For what it is worth, figs were boiled in water by early settlers and the tea sniffed into the nostrils for inflammations therein. (Figs are also demulcent in action and the reader should not be surprised to discover they are still occasionally used in cough syrups.)

Undoubtedly, there are certain marvelously balanced ingredients in carefully chosen herbs that give them their unique powers (if faithfully and *properly* used) to curb sneezing, suppress itchy or watery eyes, lessen stuffiness, open respiratory passages, reduce swelling in mucous membranes, expel or dissolve phlegm, build immunities against toxic materials, or reactivate the glands that normally produce the body's natural antihistamines. Sniffing herbs is only one pathway among many towards these ends.

While by no means a sophisticated arrangement, a Russian folk remedy for runny noses and head colds consisted of throwing a few slices of whole wheat or rye bread upon a fire and sniffing the fumes for several minutes at various times throughout the day. They also used old cotton rags for the same purpose and claimed praiseworthy results. American folk medicine practitioners were not asleep at the switch either. They claimed hay fever relief from freshly crushing and inhaling sneezeweed flowers (*Helenium autumnale*), large quantities of which have poisoned farm cattle unable to find more tasty pasturage. Besides this, they reduced dried sneeze-weed flowers to powder and sniffed it up their noses. This was said to cause sneezing and unblock the nasal passages during a head cold. The line must be drawn *somewhere* and I believe I have found the place!

SMOKING HERBS

I fully believe that smoking nonaddictive herbs for respiratory control is altogether safer than saturating the entire system with all sorts of "official" medicines, any number of which may only momentarily improve breathing while gradually undermining the kidneys, liver, stomach, or other vital organs.

When respiratory torment was my usual condition, I not uncommonly smoked my herb pipe several times daily with gratifying results—a gentle warming of the nasal passages that rapidly encouraged the expulsion of nasal-tract mucus deposits. In due time, a need to blow the nose would become urgent. It seemed best to me to let the medicinal smoke gently issue outward through the nostrils and to "swallow" it ever so often in an effort to loosen throat or chest phlegm. I learned also to avoid overpuffing so that the smoke would not overheat the nasal passages.

Not long after smoking, it is not uncommon to sense a definite opening, drying and tightening action in the nasal passages. These benefits stem from the general warmth of the smoke as well as from the stimulative, expectorant, astringent and calmative properties of the herbs. The benefits often last for quite a few hours and some herbal smokers may thus find it rewarding to smoke an hour or two before retiring because sleep is naturally more restful if there is less sinus drainage during the night.

Had it not been for the fact my system urgently needed rebuilding (which primarily involved a faithful adherence to the vital food, vitamin-mineral, detoxification, exercise, and herbal programs previously outlined) I would have relied even more heavily on the benefits of herbal smoking than I did. Undoubtedly, toxic materials are expelled during, as well as directly after, a good herbal "smoke" and I believe there is some likelihood that this therapy gradually helps the system increase its natural antibodies.

Even though herbal smoke fumes will not, I think, be unduly offensive to average respiratory sufferers (who are frequently very allergic to tobacco fumes), my tests found cigarette smokers to be annoyed by many herbal mixtures I devised. Prospective herbal smokers will, I predict, find there is no two-way street and that the same cigarette fiends who blow clouds of poisonous fumes into their faces (at a rate of several packs daily per fiend) will wax indignant when gasping respiratory victims light up only one load of saw palmetto berries, horehound, eucalyptus and yerba santa leaves. In all fairness, though, nonsmokers without respiratory disorders could be honestly disconcerted by some herbal smoking odors just as they are with tobacco, but the two-pack cigarette polluters are on mighty shaky moral ground in my humble opinion. However, among the more pleasingly fragranced herbs I've found are gum benzoin powder, anise seeds, cinnamon, cloves, lavender flowers, licorice roots, pennyroyal, peppermint, rose petals, spearmint, and white clover blossoms.

To begin with, the respiratory sufferer should consider obtaining a free-drawing pipe. From my own herbal smoking experience, I feel pipes with yellow or white bowl linings are more durable than the often quite expensive brierwood pipes. Corncob pipes are excellent and easy to clean with a little piece of paper clip wire properly straightened but the corncob is not very durable. Ladies who care not to be observed with a corncob pipe may try "rolling their own" nonhabit-forming herbal formulas in cigarette fashion and running behind a barn for respiratory benefits if fearful of censure.

Whereas commercial tobaccos are treated in order to promote rapid burning and thus increase profits, it requires a bit of extra effort to get a number of medicinal herbs to burn. One usually has to puff rather steadily to avoid relighting. Goldenrod, for example, is a quite rapid "smoke" while eucalyptus is a comparatively slow one. Moreover, some herbs such as sweet basil will seem milder and less "biting," but powdered cubeb berries (Java pepper), sprinkled in mixtures to overcome particularly difficult breathing problems, will manifest some harshness. One must thus guard against the overuse of cubeb powder in the formulas.

A few of the nonhazardous and nonhabit-forming botanicals I have successfully smoked alone or in formulas for respiratory problems are: althaea roots, anise seeds, bay laurel leaves (not to be confused with the toxic mountain laurel!), blue vervain, boneset, buchu leaves, caraway seeds, catnip, celery seeds, chamomile flowers, cinnamon, cloves, coffee grounds, coltsfoot leaves, comfrey leaves, corn silk, cubeb or Java pepper (ground or crushed), cumin seeds, dandelion flowers, elder flowers (use ONLY the dried blossoms and avoid all other parts of the elderberry bush as toxic, although the cooked berries have long been used in jams), eucalyptus leaves, fennel seeds, fenugreek seeds, goldenrod (any part), hibiscus flowers, honeysuckle flowers or leaves, hops, horehound, huckleberry leaves, hyssop (whole herb), lavender flowers, licorice roots, life everlasting flowers, marjoram, mullein leaves (or flowers), oregano, pennyroyal, peppermint, plantain leaves, red clover blossoms, redbud tree flowers, rosemary, rose petals, sage (common garden), saw palmetto berries (or more properly, I think, the berry husks), shepherd's purse, skullcap (the herb), slippery elm inner bark, spearmint, sweet balm, sweet basil, thyme (common garden), tulip tree buds (or "tulip poplar" buds), violet (common—any or all parts), white clover blossoms, and yerba santa.

As far as respiratory infirmities are concerned, there are more botanicals that can be safely smoked than can be chewed or brewed. For sundry reasons I would not *regularly* drink teas made out of blue vervain, boneset, eucalyptus leaves, hops, hyssop, lavender flowers, life everlasting flowers, pennyroyal, rosemary, sage, thyme, yerba santa, or any number of other herbs that I would not hesitate to smoke.

On occasions when I found it more convenient to smoke a single herb rather than a mixture, the following usually gave me the most excellent respiratory benefits: chamomile flowers, coltsfoot leaves, comfrey leaves, elder flowers, eucalyptus leaves, garden sage, garden thyme, goldenrod (any or all parts), mullein leaves, plantain leaves, saw palmetto berry husks and yerba santa. This is not to say by any means that I failed to receive praiseworthy relief from the other herbs I listed two paragraphs ago. From my experience, all those herbs appear to have greater or lesser stimulative, expectorant, astringent, and calmative reactions WHEN SMOKED, although they may or may not (depending on the individual herb) have one or more of these virtues WHEN BREWED as teas. In fact, herbalists have often combined herbs with differing virtues into formulas because of the great difficulty in finding a single herb that contains all the properties sought.

Peppermint, which seems to alternately cool and warm the respiratory passages, is superior in mixtures but too forceful when used alone. The same is true of regular commercial cinnamon sticks, celery seeds, cloves, poplar or tulip tree buds (*Liriodendron tulipifera*) and, of course, ground Java pepper or cubebs. As for forcefulness, even one-half pipeful of such aromatic herbs as anise seeds, calamint (or mountain mint), eucalyptus leaves, lavender flowers, marjoram, oregano, pennyroyal, spearmint or thyme smoked individually can sometimes bring a measure of quick relief to stuffy or blocked nasal passages.

However, in my testings, I found it best to blend my relatively forceful or strong herbs with those of somewhat lesser strength such as althaea roots, chamomile flowers, coltsfoot leaves, *dwarf* wax myrtle leaves (*Myrica cerifera, pumila* variety), honeysuckle blooms, mullein flowers, rose petals, sweet basil, sweet or lemon balm (*Melissa officinalis*), or violet flowers. Of course, smoking medicinal herbs will not ordinarily prove as "mild" as smoking poisonous commercial tobaccos and, unfortunately, a certain degree of harshness may often be required to relieve asthma (as when smoking Java pepper or cubebs, cloves, mullein, etc., in combination), bronchitis and hay fever attacks. Indeed, substantial mucus deposits are by no means easy to dislodge and, when one's system stands in dire need of detoxification measures, chronically blocked airways may know only gradual relief. As repeatedly indicated, patience is the cornerstone of a successful respiratory program. Just when a tortured soul feels that the struggle is hopeless, a glimmer of heavenly sunshine appears at the end of the tunnel.

Though quite strong, I always found pounded or crushed saw palmetto berries and the readily usable berry husks of specific benefit smoked alone or in numerous combinations, particularly with beech tree leaves, blue vervain, catnip, chamomile flowers, coltsfoot leaves, comfrey leaves, elder flowers, eucalyptus leaves, goldenrod, horehound, hyssop, life everlasting flowers, mullein leaves or flowers, plantain leaves, redbud tree flowers, rosemary, sage (any species), skullcap, slippery elm inner bark, sweet or lemon balm, sweet or common basil, stinging nettle (the *Urtica* species ONLY and not a number of poisonous or harmful plants locally called "nettle" due to their "armed" or "stinging" nature), violet (the herb), or yerba santa.

As for "odor modifers" or "flavor imparters," I not infrequently sprinkled in a bit of powdered gum benzoin (in particular), anise seeds, calamint, cinnamon, cloves (ground or whole), lavender flowers, licorice roots, pennyroyal, peppermint (an all-around modifier!), rose petals, spearmint, or white clover blossoms. The reader can thus concoct all manner of formulas ranging from two or three herbs to an almost unlimited number within reason and can duly invent combinations best suited to his or her individual condition. Of course, eating a meal directly after smoking, as well as brushing the teeth, should do much toward neutralizing any unpleasant smoking odors encountered, but I dare say any reader can devise a formula that will outdo the office cigar.

Anyone who is not equipped with a collection of spice rack herbs can obtain a box of Sleepytime herbal tea from a health food center for about $1.50 (in the loose pack) and try this or any number of nonhazardous original formulas. Sleepytime is not, as the name might suggest in these intemperate days, an archfiend concoction guaranteed to produce varicolored nightmares but is rather a gentle nervine formula composed of chamomile flowers, spearmint, tilia flowers, passion flowers (only a bit), raspberry leaves, hops, lemon grass, orange blossoms, hawthorn berries, skullcap and rose petals. If Sleepytime is not available, the beginner can consider testing a single basic type ingredient such as coltsfoot leaves, comfrey leaves, eucalyptus leaves, goldenrod, mullein leaves, sage (common garden), saw palmetto berry husks, thyme (common garden), or yerba santa, any one of which would convince the skeptic that here is a virtually untapped natural resource for the relief of asthma, bronchitis, and hay fever.

Who knows but what smoking coltsfoot leaves, mullein leaves or rosemary may actually be of medicinal value against a cough? Or that smoking mullein leaves will not relieve a sore throat when "swallowed" sufficiently and that a pipeful of eucalyptus leaves will do any less for labored breathing than some of the highly publicized medications of doubtful safety? This does not, however, suggest that a suspension of common sense is in order. In the case of shortness of breath suffered by heart attack victims or persistent coughs (due possibly to an obstructive growth in the throat) one should seek treatment from a competent physician. Also, certain infections, unnatural fevers of high degree, or an acute asthma attack that requires the administration of oxygen mandate the help of trained medical professionals.

During the course of my smokings, powdered benzoin gum and lavender flowers in combination seemed to alleviate itchy eyes fairly well, as did a mixture of skullcap (the herb) and elder flowers. Moreover, blue vervain, eucalyptus, goldenrod, or mullein smoked singly during hay fever attacks, had what I felt was a definitely soothing effect upon itching eyes. I hesitate somewhat to speak of it but, while smoking these and quite a few other herbs, I occasionally held a "cupped" hand over my eyebrows and allowed a small amount of the astringent herbal smoke to briefly curl upward from my nostrils into my itching eyes. I was, however, *exceedingly careful* not to overwarm the eyes. I honestly believe this unique therapeutic discovery reduced the itchy eye annoyances so associated with hay fever. To be sure, I would not have used this type of therapy even occasionally had I suffered from any loss of vision due to cataracts or from any eye ailment requiring the special attention of a physician.

But, of course, I obtained what was doubtlessly more appropriate relief from itchy eyes by merely smoking my herbs *normally*, chewing honeycomb regularly, inhaling herbal formulas as earlier described, taking a B2 (25 milligram) tablet regularly in league with my other supplements, occasionally using a natural eye remedy called

Estivin (sold in drug stores), and bathing the eyes with a soothing tea made by boiling a teaspoonful of althaea (marsh mallow) roots in about a pint of water.

I gradually, thank God, reached a time in my overall respiratory program when I could control almost any kind of hay fever encounter by merely chewing 500 milligrams or less of Vitamin C tablets on contact (or as needed). Eventually, except during pollen fallout "emergencies," I had no need to ignite my herb pipe at all.

Although most plants about us appear harmless or nearly so, a good many are toxic under certain conditions and a special few are deathly poisonous. With these things in mind, let the reader strictly *beware* of smoking stramonium or jimson weed (*Datura stramonium* or *D. meteloides*) to alleviate breathing difficulties. Stay well clear of lobelia, baneberries, henbane, bittersweet berries, English ivy, daphne berries, mistletoe berries, moonseed berries, privet berries, the various dogbanes, milkweeds of several poisonous species, oleander, star-of-Bethlehem, all larkspur species, bouncing bet, aconite or monkshood (*Aconitum napellus*), false hellebore or veratrum, foxglove, (from whence comes digitalis, a cumulative poison as well as a heart medicine), Christmas rose (*Helleborus niger*), ground rosary peas (used in bead work), death camas seeds, yellow jessamine, corn or purple cockle (a member of the pink family, the seeds of which are a cumulative poison such as one finds in so many plants including marijuana), arnica, locoweed (many species known for their cumulative toxicity), holly berries, Jerusalem or Natal cherry, matrimony vine, ground cherry or husk tomato, horse or bull nettle (*Solanum carolinense*), belladonna (this one should throw the absolute fear of God into any sane person!), yew seeds, ephedra, gamboge gum resin, grindelia or gum plant, iboga bark, jaborandi, kava kava (*Piper methysticum*), wild lettuce (*Lactuca virosa*), snow-on-the-mountain, burning bush leaves, ground castor beans, Scotch broom, dumb cane, rattlebox or rattleweed seeds (*Crotalaria sagittalis* or *C. spectabilis*), columbine berries, lily of the valley, opium poppy seeds, herb Paris, coca leaves, and copaiba resin.

The old maxim *When in doubt—Don't* should be firmly kept in mind when formulating a herbal program. The aforementioned botanicals, so far as I am concerned, are *not* to be tampered with.

I would like to assure any respiratory sufferer whose lungs are lamentably and systematically being poisoned by tobacco that nicotine addiction can be gradually conquered as follows: Load your herb pipe regularly with varying combinations of tobacco and *coltsfoot, mullein,* beech tree leaves, chamomile, eucalyptus, garden sage, marjoram, and yerba santa until such time as no more tobacco remains in the mixtures and the nonhabit-forming herbs are being smoked exclusively. As for the hacking cough so often associated with nicotine consumption, common mullein leaves are most beneficial but, tastewise, I am inclined to believe that coltsfoot leaves will remind the average user more of the adored tobacco than any other substitute.

I believe that any side effects that could accrue (and to this date I know of none) from utilizing CARE-FULLY SELECTED respiratory herbs cannot compare in harshness with some of the side effects derived from ingesting popular over-the-counter pharmaceutical miracle products or prescriptions in ever increasing doses for respiratory relief.

CHAPTER VIII
Epilogue

Quite apart from the conquest of asthma and my control over hay fever without the harmful use of popular decongestant tablets or nasal sprays, it would be remiss of me if I neglected to thank Providence for giving me complete or near complete control over such old-time adversaries as acidity; the common cold (haven't had one since early in my program!); conjunctivitis; chest pains; congestive "ear noises;" constipation; dermatitis; dizziness; earaches; fever blisters; fingernail biting; flagrant indigestion; general fatigue; hemorrhoids; insomnia (sleeplessness); "nervous spots" before the eyes; nocturnal kidney evacuations without respite; painful cracks on the lips, hands and toes; poor circulation; and "racing" pulse (as well as very high readings, without exertion, as a common body condition).

While my nervous system was considerably undermined as a consequence of several Mediterranean invasion campaigns during World War II, I must say that I have also had a providential improvement nervewise. However, I must honestly admit that, at this late time of my life, a forty-hour working week on a very stressful job is ample to-do and fermentation. And while my formerly dark brown hair is still grey as a rat (my mother's blondish hair having also turned grey early in life), I did notice with no little astonishment that my regular vitamin and mineral program triggered a gradual, albeit slight, darkening of my hair!

I am not endeavoring to "play doctor" but I do believe that the "allergy" physicians are generally on the wrong pathway and that natural (as possible) "new" or "old-fashioned" methods noted in this humble testimonial will either prevent, control or possibly "cure" a number of respiratory malfunctions publicly considered all but incurable.

I would never advocate that people stop consulting their physicians. And I would not hesitate to knock on the closest doctor's door were I bitten by a rattlesnake or mad dog. Of a truth, this treatise by a one-time asthma patient (who would, I believe, have gradually deteriorated into emphysema!) is written with no intent whatever to malign the noble practice of medicine.

Inasmuch as I have not found it *necessary* to utilize respiratory tablets, nose sprays, over-the-counter "sniffing tubes," lung sprays (or aerosol nebulizers) and other such "orthodox" medicines since February, 1973, should not our "allergy" doctors or other qualified researchers investigate some of the respiratory control therapies that were successful for me and are recorded in this manuscript? Is there any reason why ideas hatched outside a degree factory or a heavily endowed pharmaceutical laboratory should be dismissed as "crackpot" or useless?

Of course, a simple remedy that works for me may not do as much for another respiratory sufferer. However, only the Almighty knows how many people are slowly and systematically being poisoned to death with potentially harmful drugs by conscientious doctors who are unable to prevent or control the side effects that naturally accrue therefrom. Could it be that wholesome food is the only medicine that legions of wretched people need to regain their failing vigor? And is it not possible that some of our M.D.'s are "educated" beyond their own understanding?

In my personal fight against respiratory disease I came to believe that an ounce of prevention was worth a pound of cure. I was often inspired by an anonymous poem entitled "The Vicious Cycle" that says "To get his wealth he spent his health and then with might and main, he turned around and spent his wealth to get his health again!"

According to an official booklet issued in May, 1978, by the American Lung Association, a staggering total of 47,000,000 Americans of all ages SUFFER FROM ONE OR MORE CHRONIC RESPIRATORY DISEASES!

Of these, 6,000,000 reportedly have asthma and over 6,500,000 chronic bronchitis. Nicotine poisoning kills 300,000 prematurely each year and is singled out as the chief cause of chronic bronchitis and emphysema. Quite apart from tobacco-related respiratory diseases, the American Lung Association laments the horrors of *black lung* disease from breathing coal dust, *asbestosis* from inhaling asbestos fibers industrially, *berylliosis* from the inhalation of beryllium dust, and *silicosis* from breathing silica dust. Inhaling industrial dusts from mining grainite, marble and sundry metals will continue to incapacitate unknown numbers, while breathing cotton or synthetic fibers will take another toll.

After presenting what appears to be a factual report on respiratory disease (including a statement that the cost of these afflictions is estimated to be $16.5 billion annually!), the American Lung Association tells us that the toxic drugs Aminophylline and Isoproterenol are SAFE asthma medicines! The 3,500 English asthmatics said to have been killed during the sixties from inhaling too much Isoproterenol cannot testify as to the safety of this miracle drug. While the American varieties of this medication were said to have been only around one-fifth the strength of the English brand, several physicians believe Isoproterenol (or Isuprel) may interact with drugs of the cortisone family and produce potentially fatal heart irregularities. Too many allergy doctors dispense cortisone without nearly the caution they should.

Instead of the goodly sums of money collected from Christmas Seal campaigns being spent by the over two hundred American Lung Association affiliates on "orthodox" programs that cannot halfway remove (much less eliminate!) harmful respiratory drugs from the lives of most *chronic* sufferers, it would seem sensible to spend some funds on "natural" (as possible) programs based on the altered lifestyle approaches described in this book. Sickness, after all, is an outraged nature's way of punishing an offender. And some remedies are more harmful than the initial complaint.

My own providential good fortune tells me that many respiratory sufferers can *gradually* restore the body's vitality and, in so doing, *gradually* eliminate respiratory medicines the same as I have *patiently* done.

I rest my case with the profound hope that my experiences and remedies will aid other allergy or respiratory sufferers. And the hope that vital research will be stimulated as a consequence of this testimonial.

BIBLIOGRAPHY

Abrahamson, E. M., and Pezet, A. W. *Body, Mind, and Sugar.* New York: Pyramid Books, 1972.

Adams, Ruth, and Murray, Frank. *Vitamin C, the Powerhouse Vitamin, Conquers More Than Just Colds.* New York: Larchmont Press, 1974.

Alasker, Rasmus. *Conquering Colds and Sinus Infections.* Island Park, New York: Groton Press, Inc., 1967.

Alvarez, Walter C. *Live at Peace With Your Nerves.* New York: Award Books, 1958.

Atkins, Robert C. and Linde, Shirley. *Dr. Atkins' Super Energy Diet.* New York: Crown Publishers, Inc., 1977.

Bailey, Herbert. *The Vitamin Pioneers.* New York: Pyramid Books, 1970.

Bethel, May. *The Healing Power of Herbs.* North Hollywood, California: Wilshire Book Company, 1972.

Bieler, Henry G. *Food Is Your Best Medicine.* New York: Vintage Books, 1973.

Brandt, Johanna. *The Grape Cure For Cancer and Other Diseases.* Cape Town, Republic of South Africa: Creda Press, 1947. (Distributed by Mrs. E. Kellerman, 87A Hans V. Rensburgstr, Pietersburg 0700 R.S.A.)

Chapman, Esther. *How to Use the Twelve Tissue Salts.* New York: Pyramid Books, 1971.

Coca, Arthur F. *The Pulse Test—Easy Allergy Detection.* New York: Arco Publishing Company, Inc., 1977.

Coon, Nelson. *Using Wayside Plants.* New York: Hearthside Press, 1969.

Cooper, Mildred, and Cooper, Kenneth H. *Aerobics for Women.* New York: Bantam Books, Inc., 1973.

Coulter, Harris L. *Homeopathic Medicine.* St. Louis: Formur, Inc., Publishers, 1975.

Crawford, Michael, and Crawford, Sheilagh. *What We Eat Today—The Food Manipulators Vs. the People.* New York: Stein and Day, 1972.

Culpeper, Nicholas. *Culpepper's Complete Herbal.* 1662. Reprint. Slough, Bucks, England: W. Foulsham & Company, Ltd., 1975.

d'Andreta, Carlo. *Herbs and Other Medicinial Plants.* New York: Crescent Books, 1972.

Davis, Adelle. *Let's Eat Right to Keep Fit.* New York: New American Library, Inc., 1970.

__________. *Let's Get Well.* New York: New American Library, 1972.

__________. *Let's Have Healthy Children.* New York: Harcourt Brace Jovanovich, Inc., 1972.

Doyle, Rodger P., and Redding, James L. *The Complete Food Handbook.* New York: Grove Press, Inc., 1977.

Duncan, Wilbur H., and Foote, Leonard E. *Wildflowers of the Southeastern United States.* Athens, Georgia: The University of Georgia Press, 1975.

Ebon, Martin. *Which Vitamins Do You Need?* New York: Bantam Books, Inc., 1974.

Ehret, Arnold. *The Definite Cure of Chronic Constipation.* Beaumont, California: Ehret Literature Publishing Company, 1955.

Fernald, Merritt Lyndon, and Kinsey, Alfred Charles. *Edible Wild Plants of Eastern North America.* New York and Evanston, Illinois: Harper and Row, Publishers, 1958.

Finnerty, Frank, and Linde, Shirley. *High Blood Pressure.* New York: The David McKay Company, Inc., 1975.

Fredericks, Carlton. *Nutrition—Your Key to Good Health.* North Hollywood, California: London Press, 1972.

————., and Bailey, Herbert. *Food Facts & Fallacies.* New York: Arco Publishing Company, Inc., 1972.

Garten, M. O. *The Natural and Drugless Way for Better Health.* New York: Arco Publishing Company, Inc., 1973.

Graedon, Joe. *The People's Pharmacy.* New York: St. Martin's Press, 1976.

Grieve, M. *A Modern Herbal.* New York: Dover Publications, Inc., 1971.

Grimm, William Carey. *How to Recognize Flowering Wild Plants.* New York: Castle Books, 1968.

__________. *How to Recognize Shrubs.* New York: Castle Books, 1966.

Harris, Ben Charles. *Eat the Weeds.* New Canaan, Connecticut: Keats Publishing, Inc., 1973.

__________. *Kitchen Medicines.* New York: Pocket Books, 1973.

Hechtlinger, Adelaide. *The Great Patent Medicine Era.* New York: Galahad Books, 1975.

Hirshfeld, Herman. *Your Allergic Child.* New York: Arco Publishing Company, Inc., 1972.

Homola, Samuel. *Doctor Homola's Life-Extender Health Guide.* West Nyack, New York: Parker Publishing Company, Inc., 1975.

__________. *Doctor Homola's Natural Health Remedies.* West Nyack, New York: Parker Publishing Company, Inc., 1973.

James, Caudia V. *Herbs and the Fountain of Youth.* Edmonton, Alberta, Canada: Amrita Books, 1973.

Jarvis, D. C. *Folk Medicine.* Greenwich, Connecticut: Fawcett Publications, Inc., 1958.

Jones, Kenneth L., Shainberg, Louis W.. and Byer, Curtis O. *Foods, Diet, and Nutrition.* San Francisco, Canfield Press, 1970.

Justice, William S., and Bell, Ritchie. *Wild Flowers of*

North Carolina Chapel Hill, North Carolina: The University of North Carolina Press, 1973.

Kadans, Joseph M. *Modern Encyclopedia of Herbs.* West Nyack, New York: Parker Publishing Company, Inc., 1972.

Kirk, Donald, R. *Wild Edible Plants of the Western United States.* Healdsburg, California: Naturegraph Publishers, 1970.

Kirschmann, John D. *Nutrition Almanac.* New York: McGraw-Hill Book Company, 1975.

Kloss, Jethro. *Back To Eden.* New York: Lancer Books, Inc., 1971.

Knight, Allan. *Your Allergy—What to Do About It.* North Hollywood, California: Wilshire Book Company, 1976.

Kordel, Lelord. *Health Through Nutrition.* New York: Macfadden-Bartell Books, 1971.

————. *Natural Folk Remedies.* New York: Manor Books, Inc., 1976.

Kourennoff, Paul M., and St. George, Geoge. *Russian Folk Medicine.* New York: Pyramid Books, 1971.

Kremer, William F., and Kremer, Laura. *The Doctors' Metabolic Diet.* New York: Rutlege Books, 1975.

Krochmal, Arnold and Krochmal, Connie. *A Guide to the Medicinal Plants of the United States.* New York: The New York Times Book Company, 1973.

Law, Donald. *The Concise Herbal Encyclopedia.* New York: St. Martin's Press, Inc., 1973.

Lucas, Richard. *Common and Uncommon Uses of Herbs for Healthful Living.* New York: Arco Publishing Company, Inc., 1959.

Lust, John B. *The Herb Book.* New York: Bantam Books, Inc., 1974.

Macoboy, Stirling. *What Flower Is That?* New York: Crown Publishers, Inc., 1973.

Marsh, Edward, E. *How to Be Healthy With Natural Foods.* New York: Gramercy Publishing Company, 1963.

Martin, Alexander C. *Weeds.* Racine, Wisconsin: Western Publishing Company, Inc., 1972.

Meyer, Clarence. *American Folk Medicine.* New York: New American Library, Inc., 1975.

Morehouse, Laurence E., and Gross, Leonard. *Total Fitness in 30 Minutes a Week.* New York: Simon and Schuster, 1975.

Morley, Brian D., and Everard, Barbara. *Wild Flowers of the World.* New York: Crescent Books, 1970.

Morton, Julia F. *Herbs and Spices.* Racine, Wisconsin: Western Publishing Company, Inc., 1976.

Muenscher, Walter Conrad. *Poisonous Plants of the United States.* New York: Collier Books, 1975.

Ness, Maurice H. *Honey I Love You—You're So Sweet and Good to Me.* Denver, Colorado: Nutri-Books, 1966.

Novak, F. A. *The Pictorial Encyclopedia of Plants and Flowers.* London: Paul Hamlyn Publishing Group, Ltd., 1966.

Null, Gary and Null, Steve. *Herbs for the Seventies.*

New York: Dell Publishing Company, Inc., 1973.

Pauling, Linus. *Vitamin C and the Common Cold.* New York: Bantam Books, Inc., 1971.

Pokorny, Jaromir. *A Color Guide to Familiar Trees, Leaves, Bark and Fruit.* London: Octopus Books, Limited, 1974.

Powell, Eric F. W. *Kelp the Health Giver.* Rustington, Sussex, England: Health Science Press, 1971.

Preston, Harry, and Halley, Emil J. *The Natural Food Reducing Diet.* Secaucus, New Jersey: Castle Books, 1974.

Preston, Richard J., Jr. *North American Trees (Exclusive of Mexico and Tropical United States).* Cambridge, Massachusetts: The M.I.T. Press, 1973.

Quick, Clifford. *Sinusitis, Bronchitis and Emphysema.* New Canaan, Connecticut: Keats Publishing, Inc., 1975.

Régnier, Edmé. *There Is a Cure for the Common Cold.* West Nyack, New York: Parker Publishing Company, Inc., 1971.

Reid, George K. *Pond Life.* New York: Golden Press, 1967.

Robbins, Jacob John. *Asthma Is Curable.* New York: Exposition Press, Inc., 1965.

Rodale, J.I. *The Itch and What to Do Besides Scratching.* Emmaus, Pennsylvania: Rodale Books, Inc., 1971.

Rodale, Robert. *The Best Health Ideas I Know.* Emmaus, Pennslvania: Rodale Press, Inc., 1974.

Rohde, Eleanour Sinclair. *The Old English Herbals.*

New York: Dover Publications, Inc., 1971.

Rose, Jeanne. *Herbs and Things*. New York: Grosset & Dunlap, 1974.

Scully, Virginia. *A Treasury of American Indian Herbs*. New York: Bonanza Books, 1970.

Shute, Wilfrid E., and Taub, Harald J. *Vitamin E for Ailing and Healthy Hearts*. New York: Pyramid Books, 1972.

Snively, William Daniel, Jr., and Thuerbach, Jan. *Healing Beyond Medicine*. West Nyack, New York: Parker Publishing Company, Inc., 1972.

Steinhart, Lawrence M. *Beauty Through Health—From the Edgar Cayce Readings*. New York: Arbor House Publishing Company, Inc., 1974.

Stephenson, James H. *A Doctor's Guide to Helping Yourself With Homeopathic Remedies*. West Nyack, New York: Parker Publishing Company, Inc., 1976.

Taub, Harald, J. *Keeping Healthy in a Polluted World*. New York: Penguin Books, Inc., 1975

Taylor, Norman. *The Guide to Garden Shrubs and Trees (Including Woody Vines)—Their Identity and Culture*. New York: Bonanza Books, 1965.

Tobe, John H. *Proven Herbal Remedies*. St. Catherines, Ontario, Canada: Provoker Press, 1969.

Toman, Jan, and Felix, Jiri. *A Field Guide in Color to Plants and Animals*. London: Octopus Books, Limited, 1974.

Tonsley, Cecil. *Honey for Health*. New York: Award Books, 1969.

Weiner, Joan. *Get Your Health Together*. New York: Prestige Books, Inc., 1971.

Wertheim, Alfred H. *Natural Poisons in Natural Foods*. Secaucus, New Jersey: Lyle Stuart, Inc., 1974.

Winter, Ruth. *A Consumer's Dictionary of Food Additives*. New York: Crown Publishers, Inc., 1978.

Zim, Herbert S., and Martin, Alexander, C. *Flowers— A Guide to Familiar American Wildflowers*. New York: Golden Press, 1950.

______. *Trees—A Guide to Familiar American Trees*. New York: Golden Press, 1956.

INDEX